AF492061

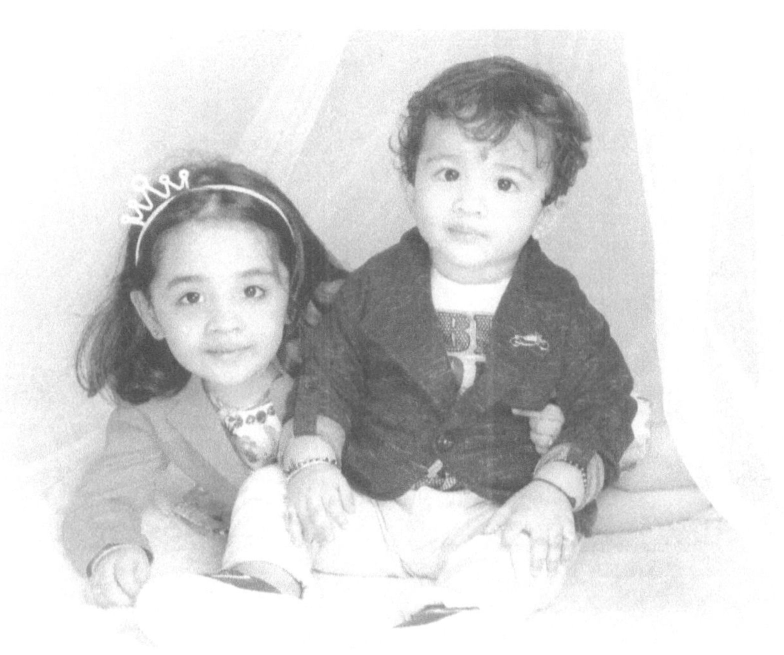

Contents

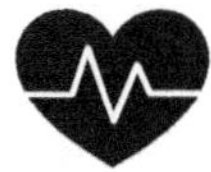

Prologue

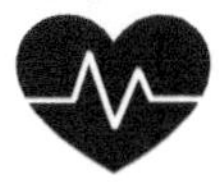

From distress to dazzle,

From hell to happiness,

From concern to contentment,

From suffering to solace,

It has all been a painful yet triumphant journey!!

His eyes were glaring, "I want us to have a child!" and my heart yearned for one too. The anticipation persisted every time we went for IVF, resulting in repeated failures mainly due to PCOD.

The crux of my challenge lay in dealing with PCOD, a condition that affects many teenage girls today, including me. PCOD, or Polycystic Ovary Syndrome, posed significant hurdles on my path to health and well-being.

The distress and suffering were unbearable. Nothing else mattered but having a child in our lives. We were determined to move mountains for our dream. We were not going to give up at any cost.

Lately, I had begun avoiding eye contact with Naresh. The best husband in the world and a wonderful human being, Naresh was now getting impatient and restless.

Every time I looked into his eyes, I felt guilty about my limitation to bear a child. We wished to have a child but I was unable to conceive. The 12-year-long journey where we did everything to have a child and repeated failures had me famished, exhausted and totally disillusioned. Inspite of being busy in our lives with business, we both felt our lives were incomplete. A void surely existed.

"When everyone can have a child, why not us?"

This is a journey of intense struggle that I wish to share with you, not to discourage but just to suggest an alternate solution. It was as if we had challenged nature that did everything to discourage us from having a child but we were adamant. I reformed my lifestyle to be able to conceive naturally.

The howl each time we failed was haunting.

I could not bear the disappointment in Naresh's eyes and the physical, mental and emotional distress I went through each time the IVF process failed. It was a self-defeating journey but we were thinking of IVF as our only choice.

Chapter 1

Jab Hum Mile

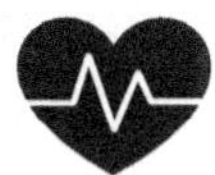

When 2 hearts meet, it is the beginning of a new life together.

The memory of getting the first glimpse of Naresh is etched in my mind; it was at our office. I vividly remember the blue crisp shirt and a helmet in his hand. Since I was a counselor, I was seated at the reception.

He looked at me, smiled and greeted me, "Good morning ma'am." I was totally unaware that someone so special was going to enter my life. They often say when we meet someone special, nature signals us. I did feel that he was special; the handsome hunk I wanted in my life. You never plan to fall in love, it just happens. Naresh was the kind of man I always dreamed of being with. Tall, handsome and chiseled body to match the killing looks. Wow!! The Salt N Pepa song, 'What a man, what a man, what a man, What a mighty good man!!' started playing in my ears.

I just loved the idea of meeting Naresh every day (at the office, of course). His personality was stunning, mesmerizing and I felt like spending the rest of my life with him. His happiness mattered and I loved it when he used to be around. Since we worked in the same office, we met every day.

On the first day of joining the office, during lunchtime I stole some glances. We colleagues used to have lunch together, so Naresh joined us. And the moment he entered the cabin the same song began playing in my mind, 'What a man, what a man, what a man, What a mighty good man!!' I was lost in my own thoughts. After a minute, I realized my behavior was that of a college kid, I shook myself and began eating my food.

We used to be busy with work most of the time so we didn't get much time to have long conversations. I started stealing glances at the office and exchanged a few conversations. That is how he slowly grew on me. I was oblivious to the fact that my colleagues had begun observing my reactions in Naresh's presence and the change in my behavior too. They guessed, "Geeta has flipped on Naresh. Yeh toh gayi!"

They didn't leave any chance to tease Naresh. "Dude she loves you!!"Naresh often reacted by saying, "Pagal, kuch bhi bolte ho tumlog." Naresh, for the kind of guy he is, kept silent. No one knew what was on his mind, neither his friends, nor me. Day by day I felt impatient. It had been some time since Naresh had joined the center. We had become friendly with each other.

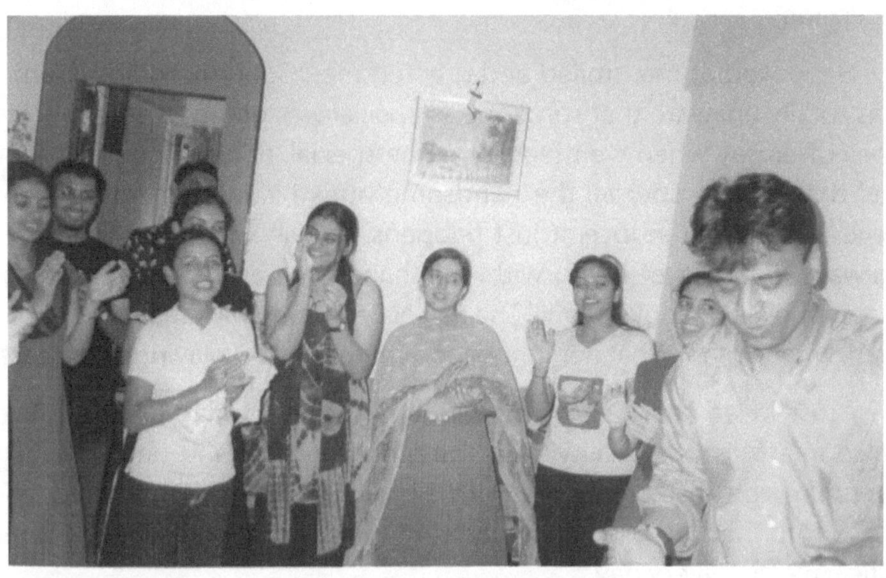

Naresh had heard me speaking about my family. He knew about my life till now; the trials and tribulations, the joys and triumphs.

A Sindhi family of 4 sisters and one brother, we lived a modest life. Till I was 17, we siblings never felt the brunt of financial challenges since my father's business was doing pretty well. But, as they say, nothing in this world is constant. Change is inherent in everything and it's also necessary for growth. My father's challenges in business changed everything for us.

Life throws challenges at strong people. When the going gets tough, the tough get going.

I began taking home tuitions to support my family. I was just 17 years old, and had just appeared for my board exams when I began earning and supporting my family. I didn't get the time to think about my life. Well aware of my responsibilities, I had the focus that was required to fulfill it. So be it; my life was different. Life threw a challenge at me and in a blink, I had accepted it.

More often it is never the severity of the situation but the denial that poses a challenge.

I didn't think twice – I knew what I had to do and never questioned anyone – not my family, nor my destiny.

Earnings weren't sufficient and too many dependents made the situation even more stressful. So, I thought of upscaling my skills. It all began when I came across a newspaper advertisement while I was searching for apt courses to upgrade my skill sets. The advertisement by CMS was about a scholarship opportunity for an IT Networking course.

Amidst a whirlwind of confusion, I found myself standing outside the CMS Ulhasnagar center. Was this the right place? Would I find the answers I sought within these walls?

Amidst the confusion that enveloped me, I sought guidance from Aruna Madam, whose wisdom and expertise offered a beacon of clarity. With a heavy heart and a mind swirling with questions, I approached her, hoping for direction and reassurance.

To my relief, Aruna Madam greeted me with warmth and understanding, her calm demeanor a soothing balm to my frazzled nerves. With patience and empathy, she listened to my concerns and offered invaluable guidance on how to navigate the scholarship exam that would determine my eligibility for discounts based on my performance.

Despite scoring only 20 out of 50 on the scholarship exam, which qualified me for a modest 20% discount, Aruna Mam, ever the diligent salesperson, presented me with a course priced at 35,000 rupees. With a clear understanding of my budget, I expressed my preference for a more affordable option.

Opting for a 15,000 rupees course over six months, after the application of the discount, brought the total to a manageable 12,000 rupees. Aruna Mam, recognizing my financial concerns, graciously worked out a payment plan consisting of easy EMIs that aligned with my budgetary needs.

Her willingness to accommodate my circumstances and tailor a solution that suited me reaffirmed my decision to enroll.

My journey started with a clear plan: two hours every morning dedicated to training, followed by college studies in the afternoons and evening tuitions.

After completing the course on IT Networking, Tiwari sir offered me a job as a trainer.

Tiwari Sir was a North Indian gentleman of shorter stature, with a simple demeanor and distinguished by his salt-and-pepper hair. He exuded warmth and approachability, endearing himself to all who crossed his path.

It was a big surprise to me. Working as a trainer for a couple of days made me realize that training is not suitable for me, because it wasn't an enjoyable experience. I resigned despite of the fact that my family needed financial support from me. I don't prefer to take up work that I dislike or don't enjoy at all. But, something better or rather the best was awaiting. I was offered the job of a counselor that was well suited to my nature and liking. I thoroughly enjoyed working as a counselor; meeting people, discussing and guiding people, knowing their strengths and weaknesses and suggesting the apt course for them became my passion. Often people were not too sure about what they needed to do with their career. Taking efforts to listen to them carefully and suggesting a suitable course was interesting.

Parents accompanied their children and sometimes looked as puzzled as their child. They did not know much about Information Technology and Networking. Those were the days when children were curious to know more about Information Technology and what career opportunities they have after completing the course. Parents just knew it's an upcoming field and there are a lot of job opportunities but failed to understand the challenges and opportunities. They weren't sure if their kid would be able to cope up with the studies and training.

It was my role to assure them about the employability of the course and that our trainers weren't only knowledgeable but would resolve all their queries. From explaining the children and the parents about the course, job opportunities to understanding their pain points, it was all about communication. I invested each day in understanding their challenges and worries to give a befitting answer. Listening carefully was a major part of my job. Only when I listened carefully could I answer their queries. All said and done, I enjoyed being at work. I loved my job.

I was offered a job at the institute. I was not too sure about how I would perform. Though Aruna madam, and Tiwari sir, the owner were confident that I would shine.

So here I was working at a CMS center at a young age trying to figure out how better I could earn – the only thing on mind being, "Would this help my family or do I need to do more?"

Anyhow, whatever I did for my family seemed little. But, today I realize its significance since attending regular college after HSC became impossible. I didn't enjoy my college days because it was a brief experience. Training, job and home tuition kept me so busy that I had no time to attend regular college. So, correspondence was the only option.

Responsibilities had barged into my life too early – well they don't take your permission.

I also had issues having my periods may be due to the stress levels and the hormonal imbalance I was experiencing. I was diagnosed with PCOD (Polycystic Ovarian Disease), which is primarily due to hormonal imbalance and genetic tendencies. Usually when girls get periods the standard menstrual cycle is when the 2 ovaries alternately release mature eggs that are ready to be fertilized each month.

In PCOD, immature or partially immature eggs are released leading to cysts - sacks of liquid thus, ovaries start swelling.

Ovaries release androgens i.e. male hormones during the menstrual cycle - but in PCOD, ovaries begin producing excessive androgens. This leads to hair loss, weight gain around the abdomen, irregular menses and fertility too in extreme cases. Well, it has no standard cure but one can change lifestyle, exercise and change the diet by consuming low sugars and carbohydrates and high fiber and protein. Polycystic ovary syndrome (PCOS) affects women of reproductive age and is a very common hormonal issue. Mostly teenage girls suffer from it. The cause is generally hormonal imbalance, irregular periods, ovarian cyst and excess of androgens. This leads to lack of ovulation and causes infertility.

Most common symptoms are unpredictable periods or absent periods.

Acne and oily skin, excess face or body hair, infertility, hair thinning, excess weight especially around the belly.

While changes were occurring in my body, I was totally focused on my duties. As Allen Saunders says, 'Life is What Happens To You While You're Busy Making Other Plans.'

Today I have reached this far in my professional life solely due to the foundation that got laid way back in **2003**

Tiwari sir trained me and by the year 2003, I had grasped the nuances of counseling. As a counselor, my efforts of guiding people led to many enrollments at the center.

People from the regional office also began appreciating me, since at a young age, I was successful in boosting sales; the enrollment figures were high, being exceptional at my job as a counselor.

While getting a grip on my life, trying to support my family on one hand and shaping my career at the other end, some wonderful moments awaited me.

Generally, colleagues used to hang out for lunch, dinner, or travel to nearby tourist destinations during weekends. But I could not join them since I had to take tuitions, study, and also manage office work along with this. I was battling multiple responsibilities. But, I desperately wanted to be with Naresh despite the fact that such trips were unaffordable. Initially, I didn't join them but later on I chose to go, since spending time with Naresh was so important to me.

Naresh was well aware of my situation and the way I was battling life on so many fronts. He had heard me share my challenges and knew my family background very well. Hardworking, dedicated, and focused - Naresh never spelled it out but had great respect for me. The way he communicated with the team, office boys, and students impressed me. People who came inquiring for various courses asked about him. They insisted that Naresh should be their trainer, only then would they enroll. They preferred him since they were assured that all queries would be resolved when he would train students. He became popular among students in a very short span of time. I loved Naresh's nature; day by day I started loving him more and more.

I became so fond of him that when he was unwell and persistently coughing, the doctor advised him to test for Tuberculosis, I fasted without water during Sankashti so that the tests would be negative. Yes, to my delight, they turned out to be negative. I was emotionally attached to him, though my love for Naresh was still unexpressed.

Naresh was extremely professional in his attitude and approach towards work. He often guided me if I had any challenges and that had me attracted even more towards him. Not only his knowledge about the subject was up to date but his communication skills were fantastic. He respected each individual and made people comfortable with his pleasing nature.

People at the center started observing that I was attracted towards Naresh and had a soft corner for him.

Since our colleagues had taken to teasing Naresh about my love for him, one day he walked up to me and said, "Would you like to go for a cup of coffee with me?"

Oh my God!! My heart melted. I was happy and nervous at the same time. I kept looking at him. Naresh was puzzled, "Hey, Geeta." I came back to my senses, "Yes, yes, sure." I knew this was the moment of my life. He is going to propose to me. I smiled and wound up my work, clearing my desk, stumbling and dropping things out of excitement. He stood there looking at the posters near the desk, pretending that he hadn't noticed me.

I packed my stuff, took my purse and we went down the office building.

"So Geeta, where do you wish to go? Any specific place?" probed Naresh.

"Hmm, any place you like." I replied immediately, smiling at him.

While traveling on his bike, I kept imagining that he would make this moment special by holding my hands and expressing his love for me. I imagined that he would say, "Geeta, I truly love you a lot and wish to be with you for the rest of my life."

For the person he was, suave and stylish, he would make me feel special. I romanticized the situation and all the wonderful moments that were awaiting me.

Though hope and excitement played havoc, I was jubilant.

We went to a local cafe and made ourselves comfortable. Naresh asked, "Hot or cold coffee?"

"Hmmm, cold coffee with ice-cream."

Once our order was through, Naresh observed I was eager to know about this sudden invitation?

Naresh opened up, "Geeta, tell me honestly, what are your feelings for me?"

I was startled, "Why, what happened? What makes you think I have feelings for you?"

Naresh was dead serious, "Geeta, I asked you first."

"Ummm…. I like you a lot and would love to spend the rest of my life with you." I answered coyly, yet honestly.

"Geeta, I have something to share with you. Please don't take me otherwise. It is great to know a wonderful person like you."

I waited, "What next, what next, just say it man." I said in my mind.

"But, I wish to marry in my community." he said firmly.

After this revelation, my mind went numb for a while. I did not react or say anything. After a whole 3 minutes of silence Naresh looked worried.

"Sorry, I hurt you." said Naresh.

I was a bit disappointed that he didn't have the same feelings for me. I never even imagined that this would be his response. This was totally unexpected. I almost felt like a fool. I tried hard to hide my true feelings of disappointment and behaved normally. But truly it was a task behaving as if nothing had happened. I had admired him for quite some time and was expecting that he had the same feelings for me. But alas, my love was one-sided.

"I replied with a heavy heart, We are friends and will continue being friends."

Relieved, Naresh said, "Uffff. What a relief. I thought I was going to hurt a beautiful, energetic and lovely girl like you."

I smiled and said, "Stop being flattery."

We laughed heartily and returned back home…

Chapter 2
Confessing Our Love

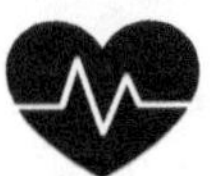

Love is all about standing by each other through thick and thin.

Naresh was firm; he wished to marry someone from his community. In the meanwhile, the work environment at the office had become extremely stressful. I had been for a job interview with my colleagues, and Tiwari sir came to know about it. He looked visibly upset and things started getting worse, day by day. Frankly, I never had a choice. My family needed my support, so I needed the job with a higher package. It had been a year at CMS Ulhasnagar but my package was still the same. I did not get a salary hike at all. So, I started searching for better options with a better pay.

One day the landline rang and my friend was on the line, "Hi Geeta, how are you?"

"I'm good." The curt answer surprised my friend.

"Though he didn't probe further. Okay, I have a job opportunity for you." he said.

"Wow, is it?"

"Yes, it's a post of a Customer Service Executive in a bank."

"I will go for it." bang came my reply.

"Well, the interviews are going on, I will send you the address." and he hung up.

He probably had no clue of how happy I was.

The next day, I went for the interview. I didn't have any idea if this was going to work out."

I was sitting at the reception when I was asked to fill out a form. I did it immediately and it was sent inside the cabin. There were a few more candidates and they looked experienced. The interviews were done within half an hour. It was my turn now. This was my first formal interview.

Knocking at the cabin door, after asking for permission to enter the cabin, I wished the Manager,

"Good morning sir!"

"Yes, Good morning. Please have a seat."

"So, Miss. Geeta. You seem to have an impressive sales background. Tell me what are your strongest points." he queried.

"I can guide, counsel, and convince people. Because I understand people and think from their point of view." I replied confidently.

The next question was confusing and a googly from the Manager.

He asked,

"So how will you convince me to commit suicide?" He smilingly asked me with the joy of having trapped me into a question that I could never answer.

I thought for a few seconds, and calmly answered, "How can I convince you about something that I'm not convinced about?"

He looked straight into me and said, "You are hired."

"Oh my God!!" I said to myself, "Is this really happening to me?"

"Thank you sir." That is all I said and went back to my office.

So, now I have a new job with a hike in salary. I was happy, and Naresh too had moved on to a company called Stream Tracmail situated at Parel. Though he didn't have any special feelings for me,

I was still hopeful that something positive will turn out. He would reconsider his feelings for me and wish to be with me. I somehow had that crazy hope that lovers do. I missed him a lot.

I worked at the new place for a few months but wasn't enjoying my job. I missed the students and the counseling part; talking to students, helping them make their choices.

Also, I was handed over a list of customers (database). My job was that of a telecaller. The whole day I called people to convince them to apply for a credit card. Most people were uninterested, so they banged the phone or were extremely rude. This continuous rejection made the job repelling and uninteresting.

Also, traveling from Ulhasnagar to Curry Road was tiring; I used to get so exhausted. Long traveling hours took a toll on my health too. Though the work environment was pleasant, and I had become friendly with my colleagues and enjoyed their company, the work itself was drop dead boring.

I continued with the routine and hoped I could just get to do something better that I could truly enjoy. This job was just not meant for me. Though I didn't have much of a choice, so I simply continued.

One day I received a call from Sriram Ramamurthy, the regional Manager of CMS, "Geeta there is an opening for a counselor's post at the Thane CMS. Wish to join?"

I didn't believe this. This was a golden chance to go back to my old profile that I enjoyed thoroughly.

"Yes, will apply and thanks a lot for informing me." I humbly answered.

When I went there at CMS Thane it felt like home. I was rather cut out for the job. Though it wasn't that easy to cope with the Center Manager. But, I consoled myself,

"Geeta, you love the job. It is stressful and the Manager is tough to work with. But, this is your favorite work profile. Things will change."

With this hope and belief, I patiently kept working. Day by day stress was adding up. I didn't want to quit though. Suddenly, the Center Manager and the whole team quit to open their branch at Borivili.

"What a relief!" I sighed. But the next thought was, "How will the center run?"

The owner Dr. Ajay Naik urged me to run the center, and since he was a doctor, he was not too involved in running and managing the center. He needed someone whom he trusted to manage the whole show. It was a challenge, but I decided to take it up. The stress didn't lessen. To hire a team, train them, counsel students, keeping a tab on the sales figures, business reviews, meetings, etc. I learned a lot about leadership, business, and management. Since I was the center head and the counselor's position was vacant, I asked my sister Pooja to join as a counselor.

One day while being busy working at the center the phone rang. I avoided the call for some time but since it rang persistently, I picked up the call.

I said, "Hello, Geeta here from CMS Thane."

The person on the other end said, "How are you Geeta?"

I instantly recognized the voice, "Oh, hi Naresh. What a pleasant surprise. I'm doing well. Thank you, how are you?"

"Yes, I'm fine. How are things at the center? All well?"

"All is well at your end. Where are you these days?"

"I have got a job at Stream Track Mail in Parel and doing quite well. Happy with the new opportunity and enjoying my job."

He called at the right time. We didn't have a CCNA Trainer at Thane CMS and he was CCNA certified trainer, so I requested him to visit the center and train students once a week as a visiting faculty. I knew Naresh's approach, skill, and knowledge were up to the mark.

Naresh heeded to my request of visiting the center to teach our students. Though he had a well-paid job, he had accepted my offer to visit the center as a faculty. Destiny had brought us together again. I thought maybe something was in store for both of us.

I was so happy that he agreed to visit the center because now I would be meeting him and spending at least some time with him. Though he came from a financially strong background, Naresh seemed to be grounded, dedicated, hardworking and wasn't pampered at home. He was extremely disciplined and focused about his career. His sincere approach to work and overall attitude towards life had me attracted to him. I longed that he would reconsider my proposal and would say yes. As of now, my love for Naresh was one-sided.

At home front, things were brewing.

My parents were looking out for a good match for my elder sister Seema. Though she was tall, fair and extremely beautiful, finding the right match became challenging. She got a proposal from a person whose marriage had been canceled. The family wished the marriage to be held in a month's time. Now this was a herculean task. We had to make quick arrangements and for all this, we needed a good amount of money. In Sidhi families, marriages are grand and above all, the girl's family has to spend a lot to keep everyone happy.

At the Thane branch as a Center Manager, my pay was good enough that enabled me to get my sister married. A proud achievement for me and moments of fond memories. Fond memories never fade; they brighten up your life to keep inspiring you.

Everyone was pretty taken aback by the arrangements since most of our friends and relatives knew about our financial challenges. I ensured that all rituals and traditions were followed and the bridegroom's family was happy with no room to complain. To cover the entire expenses and not leave the bridegroom's family complaining was a massive challenge.

Even though my sister was so beautiful, finding a match for her was so tough. While I was so short and not as pretty as her, then how could I get a suitable match within our community? All these questions hovered over my mind and I became totally negative about the idea of getting married.

On the day of the marriage, I realized getting married in the Sindhi community was truly a task. It is a ritual that when the bridegroom gets out of the car a Shagun (a ritual of gifting money) has to be given. I didn't manage to arrange for it and my brother-in-law was hell-bent on receiving an amount of Rs. 5000/-. At the last moment, we somehow arranged for that as well. This created unnecessary tension. It made me feel miserable about getting married in the Sindhi community.

Frankly, that was the point where I decided to never marry in a Sindhi family due to these oppressive traditions. In fact, for a while, I felt marriage itself was unnecessary if it would involve so much tension.

I thought, "Why do I have to go through such an ordeal just to be married? We marry for love, care and companionship. These reasons are true for both every man and woman. Then, why only the bride's family should be spending for the marriage. I could never understand this logic and it irritated me to no extent.

But, I was delighted to see Naresh present at all the functions from Mehendi to Haldi to Bidai. All through the marriage, Naresh was there to help me and support me. I grew fonder of him and felt assured that he is just the right person for me. If Naresh could be such a great friend, and be there to support me unconditionally, then surely he could be a doting husband as well.

Conversations over lunch breaks and office picnics made him quite aware about my family background and the fact that I was working hard for my family. He always wanted a family-oriented girl. Naresh wondered if at such a young age, I could have shouldered so many family responsibilities, then I would certainly be a great wife. Even while everyone had finished shopping for my sister's marriage, I hadn't shopped for myself since we had no money left after all the marriage expenses. In fact, Naresh then bought a dress for me and that gesture changed everything. I was floored. Well, this gesture was the final endorsement to my belief that Naresh could be a doting husband.

One fine day, Naresh asked me out and we went to the same coffee shop where he confronted me about my feelings for him. When we were seated and halfway through sipping the coffee, he said,

"Geeta, will you be my counselor for life."

I was quite taken aback, couldn't decipher what he was trying to say.

"You stupid girl, he is proposing to you," said my mind.

"Of course, I would love to. Frankly, I have been waiting for so long."

I paused and shared with him my biggest worry. Now I would enter a new life. But at the back of my mind, I was worried for my family. Since my siblings were too young, who would shoulder the responsibility of the family?

So, I responded out of worry, "But, even after marriage I should be able to support my family."

To which Naresh answered immediately, "We will support our family. I'm part of the family now."

I was so relieved and happy that Naresh understood my challenge. Contrary to the Sindhi community, which was strictly patriarchal and believed that a girl's family should be the one always giving gifts or money, here Naresh agreed to stand by me and support my family. This probably was one of the most important reasons as to why I was reassured about Naresh being my right choice as a life partner.

Naresh confessed, "It is not going to be easy for my parents to accept a girl outside our community. But I will convince them."

Chapter 3

Destined to be Together

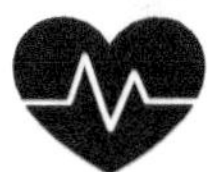

Lovers depart only to meet again and grow fonder.

Our courtship began and on weekends we visited a place called Durgadi Fort at Kalyan. It is a wonderful spot with lush greenery, cool breeze and peace. It is a kind of space where we enjoyed the serene silence and each other's company as well.

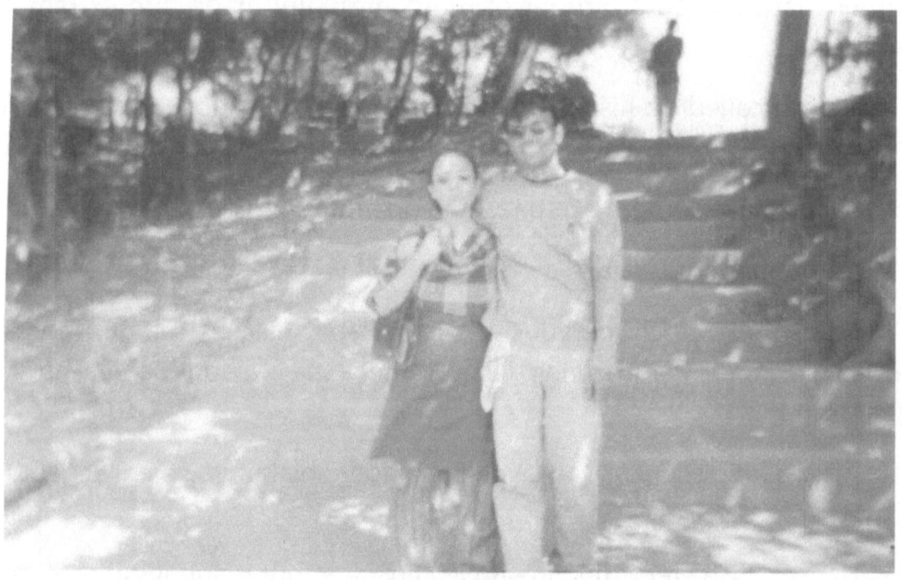

We often spent time at a local cafe and a garden called Durgadi talking for hours and sometimes sitting close to each other silently. I treasure those times; unforgettable memories that are close to my heart.

Weekdays we met at Thane station and our love bloomed as we couldn't get enough of each other. We longed to get over the phone to talk for long hours and watch movies. For so many years I had been so busy focusing on supporting the family that I paid least attention to my looks or dressing. But now I wished to dress up well, wear makeup, look trim and beautiful. Life changed completely after I started dating Naresh. I loved getting dressed for Naresh. He was the reason for my happiness.

Since we were meeting every day, both were doubly assured about the fact that we wanted to spend our lives together.

We dated for 2 years and then finally decided to open up the news to our parents. This was not going to be easy but we decided that it was time to disclose the secret we had kept for long.

It was tough for Naresh to open up to his dad about me, so he chose to speak to him over the phone and inform about us. Telling his father that he liked a girl out of the community made him extremely anxious.

Naresh called up his father on the landline and spoke in Marathi to his father,

"Dad, I have something to talk to you about."

Dad impatiently said, "Yes, tell me?"

Naresh, extremely nervous, replied, "Baba mala ek mulgi avadte. I love a girl. Pan ti Marathi nahi, ti Sindhi ahen- she is a non-Maharashtrian, she is Sindhi."

After a long silence, Dad said, "Bara, does she know we are Schedule Caste?"

Naresh answered, "Yes, she is well aware about it and it's acceptable to her."

Back in 2004 inter-caste marriages were not too acceptable and this alliance would not get anyone's support. In fact, in the Sindhi community, marrying out of caste was like being a rebel. My marriage would not be accepted by anyone, neither from my family, nor relatives. The narrative wasn't different for Naresh. His parents would not accept either. Being the only child they had a lot of expectations from him. They certainly wished for a girl from their community.

After work, when Naresh returned home his father conveyed his apprehension.

He said, "I'm not happy with your decision and I don't want a girl outside the community as my daughter-in-law. Also, are you aware of the challenges that you will face in this kind of a marriage? People from our community will not like this and will not invite you for any community functions. They won't support you. There is a strong opposition within the community for an inter-caste marriage. Have you thought about all this Naresh, I think you are making a hasty decision. Rethink son. If you ask me, it's a completely wrong decision."

For me all the opposition didn't matter. I loved him dearly and still do. It was the same for Naresh as well.

On learning his father's disapproval, Naresh stopped having food and insisted that he would marry me or never marry at all. Meanwhile, he got great proposals for marriage, which he was totally disinterested in. He was adamant and quit talking to everyone in the family. Ultimately, Naresh's mother convinced his father and urged him to stop being so rigid.

She explained, "Let us get him married to Geeta as he will not listen to us. We should be happy and accept his choice. Our son's happiness should be ours too. He is adamant but I think he is confident about his choice."

I was totally unaware of these things. I came to know about it later after his parents agreed.

Now it was my turn to reveal my choice. I had no one but my elder sister Seema, so I confessed about Naresh to her over a call.

"Seema, I want to share something with you."

"Yeah, tell me what's up?"

"I love a guy and wish to marry him," I confessed.

Seema screamed out of joy, "Oh, really!! Who is he?"

Hesitantly I shared, "His name is Naresh Khandare."

"Wait a minute, he is not Sindhi?" she almost yelled rudely.

I said in a low voice, "Di, I want you to convince mom and dad about Naresh; he is a Maharashtrian."

Seema vehemently opposed, "Forget convincing mom and dad. I will not even come for your marriage. The decision is all yours but I won't support it. If my hubby comes to know about your choice, he will stop me from visiting our home. So please, Geeta, don't bother me."

I was shocked by her reaction. Now only Pooja, my younger sister could help me. I asked Pooja to tell my parents about Naresh and when she ultimately broke the news, my mother was furious. I had told my family that I wasn't interested in marriage at all. Now I was asking for permission to marry a Maharashtrian boy. She could not believe my bold decision.

She yelled, "You weren't interested in getting married, and now you are so shamelessly telling me that you want to marry a Maharashtrian boy. Do you know the repercussions of this decision? The community will not only oppose us, they will chastise us. Oh God, why didn't I die before hearing this decision of yours. We educated you all not to make these wrong decisions in life. We hoped that education would make you wise but, instead, it has made you stupid and shameless."

She fired at me a lot and ultimately refused to talk to me. My father has always been calm so he didn't react much. Though being at home was tough, it felt like we were mourning. It was like living in hell. No one spoke and everyone looked disturbed. Unable to understand where all this will lead to, I kept mum. I didn't speak to anyone. It is tough to walk the untrodden path, but if you believe in yourself and the choices made by you, nothing can stop you.

Once again I had acted like a rebel, not purposely but it was destined to be like that. I probably didn't choose to be a rebel but my choices were that of a non-conformist.

My mother knew very well that this decision won't be supported by anyone from our community. She was worried about facing the community. At this juncture, I felt that I had taken a decision that would not be supported by anyone at all and it was rather the biggest challenge I had ever faced in my life.

No one seemed to be happy. But it didn't matter to both of us. We gave some time to our families to absorb the challenge and waited for them to accept it. We were not going to give up.

We came from different backgrounds, and cultures. A fusion of this kind was unimaginable for my and Naresh's family. It has so happened that I have always chosen to follow my heart. In doing so, I have been the first person to try things that no one ever had in my family. I have been the first one to do a job in our family, the first one to marry outside our caste and the first one to go for IVF. Nonetheless, I don't regret any of my decisions. It has all been a learning experience and I have grown tremendously as a person.

Life has always something more to offer you. But, are you ready to welcome it?

Do you embrace change and growth? Yes, I did and still do! As we both were busy working at our respective jobs, me at CMS and Naresh at Stream Tracmail, I saw a newspaper advertisement that CMS was offering a franchise for Kalyan center. The first person I thought of was Naresh to partner with for establishing a franchise.

He was not only knowledgeable but also responsible, professional, disciplined, and humble by nature. Naresh knew the subject well and students adored his style of teaching.

I immediately called up Naresh and told him, "Hey, you know I just came across an advertisement that CMS is offering a franchise for Kalyan. I strongly believe we can start a franchise together. I'm well aware of the functioning of the center, the sales part and you have technical knowledge. What do you think?"

Let us meet and discuss. The next day he disclosed,

"Well Geeta, I have an offer from Shanghai. So, once I get the VISA, I will leave India. I wish to go. I will be leaving soon, Geeta."

I just couldn't believe my ears. Was this for real? I was not going to be able to meet him? My mind just shut and so did my ears to what he said next. The last words I heard were,

"I will be leaving soon Geeta."

I kept weeping continuously and uncontrollably. Naresh was going so far away from me; I didn't want to lose him at all. I couldn't imagine my life without Naresh. He was the backbone of my life.

Later, I tried convincing him "We can have our own branch here itself in Kalyan and flourish the business. Why travel all the way there? We can have our own set up here; it's much better than working for someone else."

Naresh thoughtfully said, "I have already planned everything Geeta."

I was totally disappointed and disheartened.

Life is not what we plan. It is full of surprises and a bundle of magic. No matter how much you plan, life will throw a googly at you. I didn't know what was in store for us.

In the next few days, things changed completely. Naresh's father had chest pain and insisted that Naresh should not leave India. Since he was the only son, Naresh's parents wanted him to live with them.

That is how life is; full of surprises. So, just within a week, Naresh called me to say,

"Geeta, I think we should go ahead with your plan of setting up a branch. I'm all for it. Since I have decided not to go to Shanghai, let's plan for a new center."

My happiness knew no bounds. I had waited for this day and now it was a reality.

So, eventually, Naresh stayed back in India for us to work together.

After a few days, we had begun planning the setting up of our branch.

With Naresh's funds, training knowledge and my sales skills, we were able to begin a franchise on 11th April 2005. We took a space near the station that needed to be furnished appropriately. Naresh finished his night shift where he worked at Parel and came to the center in the morning to keep a close watch on the setting up of the center. Till the center started full-fledged, Naresh was managing his job and setting up of the center. He worked extremely hard from the day we decided to start the franchise.

Once the center set up and students started enrolling we both left our respective jobs and focused only on our business. Both of us dedicatedly worked to build the business. Naresh managed the training part and I was focused on sales. We did well for us and proved our mettle. We did better than even the South Mumbai centers. Also, I think it was best for our relationship, since we were together a lot; spoke, discussed and grew together.

Nonetheless things did settle in our respective families. His and my family agreed, not too willingly, but they did. Kundalis didn't match and I was tense again, but the issue was resolved after agreeing to change my name as per the astrologer's advice. Thank God, this issue got resolved immediately without much fuss.

Naresh's mother hosted a ceremony at our office.

25th November 2005, we got married and I was the happiest person on this earth. I couldn't believe that my dream of getting married to Naresh had come true. My eyes brightened up and it was pretty evident that I was jubilant and my happiness knew no bounds.

I dressed up like a typical Maharashtrian bride with green bangles, hair adorned in typical gajara (flowers) and a pretty Mangalsutra, and heavy gold jewelry, which I totally loved.

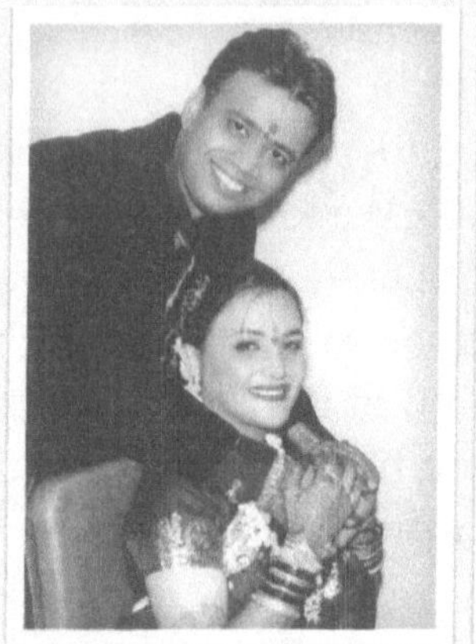
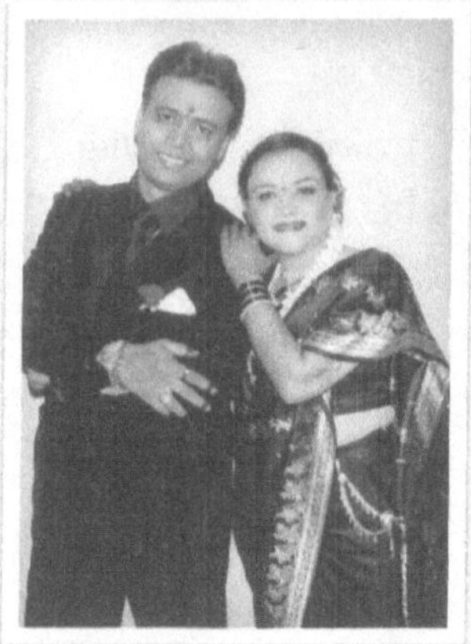
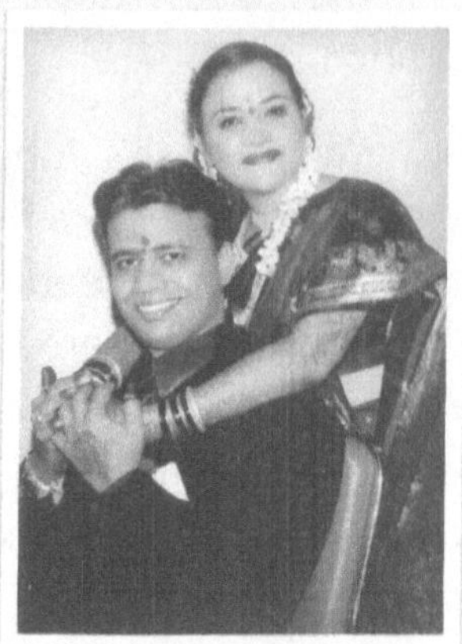

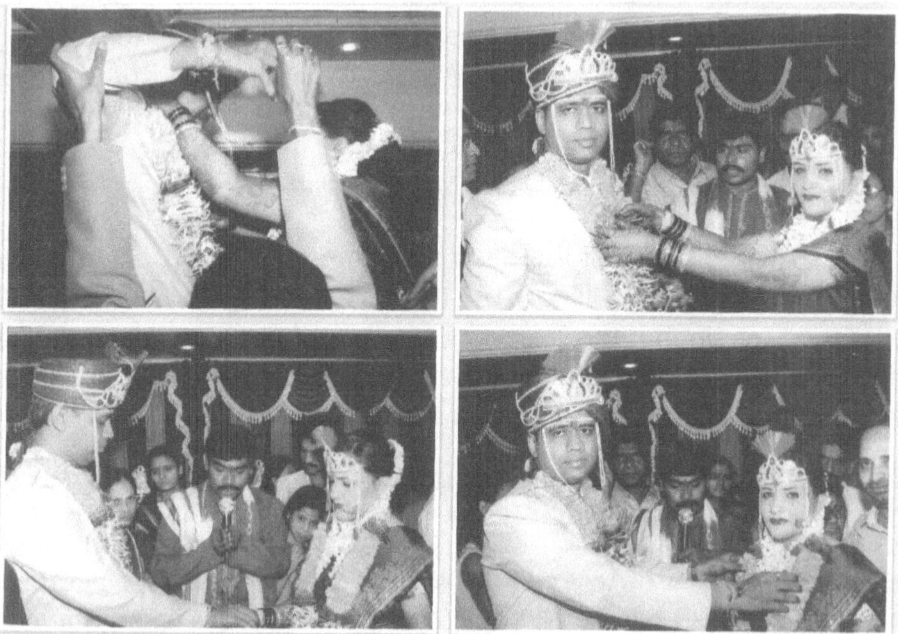

It was a grand ceremony and everyone was amazed by the grandeur. I was dressed in a green saree with delicate and exquisite embroidery. There were 200 guests from Naresh's circle but very few people (only 25 guests) attended the wedding from my side. Though the entire CMS staff was present at the wedding and ensured all the arrangements were made from decorating the car with flowers to bursting crackers.

I wasn't nervous or fearful about having an inter-caste marriage. Finally, the man of my dreams was now my life partner, and it was the beginning of a new life together.

After marriage, we had to visit so many temples that I lost my patience. I felt so exhausted moving from one temple to another and longed to go back home. Once we returned home, it was time to go for our honeymoon. My father-in-law had booked our tickets to Ooty and a villa as well. This was the first time I traveled by flight, and it turned out to be the most exciting experience.

Being with Naresh in the lovely hill station was mesmerizing. Nature seemed to be at its best, and we could not get enough of each other. The mist spread all over the hills made us feel as If we were in the clouds. The lush green carpet was nestled with trees all over the place. We were in each other's arms, cuddling and making love. It was a treat to go for long walks down the lanes and in parks. I had to pinch myself so many times to assure myself that I wasn't dreaming. Here I was with the love of my life in a paradise filled with love. After a week of living in a dreamy world, now we were back to Mumbai - facing the practical challenges of the real world.

When I started living with Naresh, things weren't that simple, though I was ready to adjust. The challenges of having an inter-caste marriage slowly unfolded. Naresh's family was hardcore non-vegetarian, and I was a pure vegetarian. It was difficult for me to adapt. The first year of marriage was tough due to the difference in eating habits. Their cuisines varied from ours, and the preparations were different.

On the first day at the breakfast table, I was served kheema pav, and I lost my appetite. I had never had non-veg food in my life. I couldn't eat much, and everyone got upset. Even when I was served Kadhi, it wasn't like our regular Sindhi Kadhi that I ate at home.

I just poured a few drops of the Kadhi on the rice on my plate and began eating. My mother-in-law could understand my challenges. In fact, Naresh felt a bit upset and angry since I wasn't able to adjust. I couldn't even make tea since I had started working at a young age.

Cooking was not my cup of tea. Naresh started becoming a bit stern with me, and his approach toward me changed. My health began deteriorating, and I started doubting my own decision of marrying outside the community. Loving each other is different from living with each other.

Life comes in a package, and we have to accept it in totality. While Naresh was a bit tough on me, my mother-in-law took care of me and introduced non-vegetarian dishes into my diet, bit by bit, in smaller portions. She has always been extremely supportive and always stood by me.

I could have chosen to continue eating vegetarian food, but I thought food is something that binds people together and connects them. So, if I had to truly become a part of Naresh's family, I had to dissolve completely into them. My only concern was that he and his family should be happy. The rest was insignificant.

I strongly believe that I did not just marry Naresh, but it was an alliance of 2 families, and I had to be a part of the family. Being married to Naresh meant accepting every aspect of his life, and family being the vital part. He knew my thoughts about marriage and the value system I believed in, thus he chose me. During my sister's marriage, he observed how well I had embraced everyone and faced the challenges. So his answer had turned from 'no' to 'yes' to my proposal. As days passed by, we started being comfortable with each other, and it all looked like one happy family. Also, the business was doing very well with continuous enrollments and high profits.

Chapter 4

The First Step to Motherhood

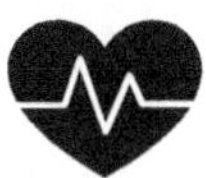

Dreams are the fountainhead of life. They are the reason for our existence and inspire us to never give up.

In these 2 years of courtship, I had realized his love for kids. His happiness is all that I pray for and can go to any limits to see him happy. At home, everything seemed to be cordial. My in-laws appreciated the way I successfully handled the business and managed to be a great daughter-in-law. But I knew one thing for sure, if I would give birth to a child, my in-laws would pamper me a lot and my husband would also love me even more. I longed for affection and attention, which was missing in my life, since I couldn't give them a child.

I also wished to escape from the responsibilities of cooking and managing the kitchen, which I was totally new to. After having a child I would probably get an escape. Actually, I was young and immature so, these things mattered to me a lot and these thoughts fogged my mind.

This desperate thought of mine made me visit the doctor immediately after marriage in December 2005. My husband was aware of my PCOD problem before marriage. My periods were irregular and I used to bleed for 15 to 20 days at a stretch. We consulted a gynecologist based in Ulhasnagar, Dr. Jeswani. Our business was shaping up and my presence mattered. Since Dr. Jeswani was available during my office hours, so it was a challenge to visit the doctor. Thus, I had to compromise on my work.

I still remember the first visit at Dr. Jeswani's clinic. We were excited, yet nervous and kept thinking about what would be the doctor's reaction.

We reached the clinic in the afternoon and were called inside his cabin. After looking at us visibly nervous Dr. Jeswani said,

"Good afternoon. You can relax first."

She offered a glass of water to us both. We took a sip, felt a bit okay and started sharing our apprehensions.

"Doctor, I have PCOD and it's a challenge for me to conceive. Do you think I will be able to conceive naturally?"

She asked a few questions and said,

"We have to trigger ovulation and increase the chances for pregnancy."

She put me on pills that triggered ovulation and increased the chances of pregnancy. Every month I had a routine internal sonography done to check if I was ovulating. It was stressful; hope is such a positive word but for me, to be in anticipation every month was killing me. The wait got longer and longer. Only disappointment came our way.

Every time I went for a sonography, nothing worked out for me. We gave up on this treatment after repeated failures

By that time, my friend had delivered a baby boy at Venkatesh Hospital, Kalyan. We went to see her there and also met her doctor. We were impressed by Dr. Venkatesh Vaidya's degrees and qualifications that he had earned from London. Thus, we began consulting Dr. Venkatesh Vaidya. He advised a Laparoscopy. It was done to identify the abnormalities that might be hindering my pregnancy.

Dr. Venkatesh asked Naresh also to get tested and his reports were excellent. So it got confirmed that I needed to undergo treatment and I had faced an issue.

We were desperately trying these treatments without informing our parents. Since we could not open up to them about the fact that my periods were irregular. It was hardly a year since we were married and we were struggling with this situation. All the test results were normal, he put me on pills to trigger ovulation and we were indicated by the doctor to be sexually active during particular dates. This went on for 6 months rendering no results.

The failure made us miserable. Failure after failure, things got from bad to worse. There was no respite, despite of approaching another doctor. A period of 6 months went in anticipation, tension and anxiety. The physical stress on a woman is always present due to hormonal changes, and menses. But the most neglected aspect of a woman's health is her emotional and mental health. She goes through so much, and it's taken for granted that she will handle it somehow. It is as if she doesn't have a choice and she better learn to manage pain both, physical and emotional.

Why? Because we are conditioned to believe that women have the tenacity, patience and strength to handle these challenges. Anyways, she was born with it so she should be able to face it. Then in what way is a woman any less than a man? Why do men get paid more than women? These thoughts hover my mind but, I've yet to get a valid and convincing answer.

Let's get back to my journey.

I felt the void in my life because both Naresh and I wanted a child desperately. I felt so helpless and guilty at times that I couldn't give birth to a child; I couldn't make my hubby and his family happy. Every month my mother-in-law asked me if I got my periods with the hope that I could have missed them, but she was totally unaware that I had PCOD, so I missed my periods due to that and not because I was pregnant. Ultimately, we did inform our parents that I was suffering from PCOD.

My sister-in-law got married after me yet, she gave birth to a child and I was still facing challenges in conceiving. She moved in for a few months with us and was pampered a lot by my in-laws, while I felt neglected and became more desperate for a child. I also longed for their affection and appreciation. And I knew that I could not make them happy as I couldn't give them a grandchild.

Meanwhile, the doctor now suggested that since the Laparoscopy reports are normal, we can go in for IUI.

I suffered from PCOD so the doctor advised us Intrauterine Insemination IUI. It's a treatment for infertility where the sperms are placed in the uterus by injecting them into a woman's uterus to facilitate fertilization.

IUI is a treatment given for unexplained infertility and women who have issues in ovulation like PCOD.

It is a part of Assisted Reproductive Technology or ART and less invasive as compared to other methods. So, now the doctor tracked my natural menstrual cycle and controlled it with fertility medications. The doctor's team closely monitored the ovulation through ultrasound and blood test to know the timing when the egg releases.

When the IUI procedure was to be done, Naresh's semen was collected so that they could separate the healthy sperm from other components. This process we were told is called sperm washing.

Then we were called for the IUI procedure at the doctor's clinic. I was made to lie down on the examination table just in the same way when the pelvic is examined. A speculum (medical device) was inserted into my vagina. This process was done to get access to my cervix. Later a thin tube or catheter was inserted through the cervix to get into the uterus.

Now the doctor took the sperm sample to load it into the catheter and vigilantly injected it into the uterus. This took a few minutes and it made me a bit uncomfortable. I was told to lie down and rest for 15 to 20 minutes and then sent home. We had to go back home and wait for the results. After 2 weeks of the IUI procedure, a pregnancy test was performed. The success rate of IUI varies and depends on various factors like the causes of infertility, quality of the sperm and the woman's age. In our case, I was not too old and the sperm quality was good too. The first time we went for IUI we didn't get a positive result, so we tried the second time and kept trying.

When repeated efforts failed, the doctor called us to meet him. We went to the hospital and were contemplating his response. We were worried about why he had called us over. We had an appointment at 3pm but we reached the hospital an hour earlier out of anxiety. There was a big question mark on our faces and we couldn't stand the suspense anymore.

Ultimately, Dr Vaidya called us in his cabin at 3pm sharp. We both looked vividly worried and waited for his advice.

Dr Vaidya said, "This procedure was repeated 6 times without any positive results. Now that we know medicines didn't work nor did IUI, we should opt for IVF."

I said with a heavy voice, "No doctor", and just broke down crying and didn't know why nature was being so ruthless with me – our struggle didn't seem to end nor our agony.

It was a testing time and the doctor consoled us by saying, "Geeta you are crying now. But, think about it. After giving birth to a child, you will be so happy. The joy will be boundless." Now we had to choose to go for IVF, a considerably rare solution in those days.

I had an impending question for the doctor, "If I give birth to a girl child, will she also have to go through this agony?"

My doctor empathetically replied, "Don't think so much, Geeta. Your baby will carry Naresh's genes too. Above all, PCOD patients have high chances of conceiving through IVF." I felt a bit relieved, but not too sure about how this new procedure was going to work out for us. We were made to sign documents, and then I was given fertility medications to stimulate the ovaries and trigger the formation of eggs. The development of follicles or the sacs that contain eggs was closely monitored through ultrasound scans and hormone level tests.

The doctor was happy that I was responding well since the amount of eggs produced was good. This is how PCOD patients respond to IVF; either they produce too many eggs (excessive) or too less (deficient).

The procedure then progressed when the follicles became mature; a trigger shot of human chorionic gonadotropin (hCG) was given to induce final egg maturation. After 36 hours, I was sedated and a minor surgical process was conducted called the egg retrieval. In this procedure, a thin needle was inserted into the ovaries through the vaginal wall to retrieve the mature eggs.

When the eggs had to be retrieved, the pain was excruciating. The eggs were produced in large numbers, and retrieving them caused me unbearable pain. Well, on the same day, Naresh's semen sample was taken and processed at the lab to collect the healthy ones. This procedure is similar to the one done during IUI.

As all this was going on, we were both nervous. Now, it was time to combine the retrieved eggs with the chosen sperm in a culture dish in the laboratory. The fertilized eggs are called embryos. These embryos are cultured and monitored in the lab for around 6 days.

We were eager to know the result, and we were told that the quality of the embryos was being assessed. The healthiest embryo is then transferred. Some good quality embryos were also frozen for future use.

Now the real procedure was to be conducted. The embryos were transferred into my uterus, which was a simple procedure.

I was part of the first batch of IVF there at the center. There were around 15 of us in the first batch, and we hadn't met earlier. But, when the embryos had to be transferred, we all met since it was done on the same day for all patients. Most of the ladies were in the age group of 35 to 45.

I was the youngest; everyone said they were taken aback that despite being so young, I opted for IVF. I still could go for a normal pregnancy. But I was desperately waiting to be a mother, and I knew very well the reason for our happiness.

We trusted the process, the way we were told, as we both wanted a child. And I was asked to rest for 2 hours and then sent home. Now I had to rest for 15 days, and then there would be a Beta-hCG test done that would determine if I was pregnant.

When we went home, I felt uncomfortable. I was on total bed rest, and then things started getting worse. My stomach began to bulge.

After a day or 2, I had breathlessness. I was so restless that my husband felt scared and worried.

We went back to the same doctor. He examined me and asked, "What is happening?"

I replied, "Doctor, I feel very restless. I can't breathe properly."

The doctor asked, "When did you last pass urine?"

"I'm trying to pass urine, but I can't."

"I'll be back soon," said the doctor and rushed out.

He made me lie down in the operation theater for a long time, and my BP was closely monitored. They put me on a wheelchair, which I resisted, but the doctor kept insisting. I had no inkling what was going on with me or the treatment. It all seemed like a mystery about me, my health, and my dream of having a baby.

What next?

Chapter 5
Brutal Truth and Agony

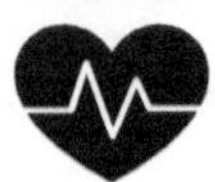

The practicalities of life are brutal; agony becomes an inseparable part of life as destiny chalks a different path.

After some time, I realized I was being shifted to Bombay Hospital. I was admitted to the ICU. My body was swollen, it was all beyond control. My vagina, stomach, legs and entire body had started slowly swelling a lot. I was breathless and restless. I was under observation in the ICU under Dr. Indira. She revealed that I was suffering from hyperstimulation[1] that rarely happens during IVF. OHSS is a complication that occurs in few patients during in vitro fertilization (IVF) and some other fertility treatments that include ovarian stimulation. OHSS is a result of ovaries overresponding to medications. It leads to enlarged ovaries and other symptoms.

When we asked the doctor, she explained that medications used to stimulate the ovaries are given. These medicines induce the development of multiple follicles in the ovaries. But women suffering from PCOD are prone to OHSS.

Ovarian hyperstimulation syndrome (OHSS) Mild OHSS is common during IVF, and 33% of women suffer from it. While moderate or severe OHSS occurs among 1% of women. I was rather unlucky to face this issue. My family was tense and restless. My in-laws were worried about what had happened to me and why I was admitted to the hospital. At that juncture, we told them about the fact that we had opted for IVF since I was suffering from PCOD.

Though they had some hope when Dr Indira mentioned,

"I think she is expecting. The chances of pregnancy among women facing hyperstimulation are pretty high."

We were hopeful and happy that it is going to be worth the trouble.

Being in ICU feels lonely; it's an isolation unit, I would say. I was alone, and no one being around made me miserable. We all need our loved ones around when we are unwell, when we are in physical or mental agony.

Pain cannot be handled alone, but unfortunately, we all are forced to be alone when in pain because your pain cannot be felt by others. You and only you have to endure the share of pain in your life.

Though undeniably my husband was part of this journey that we traveled; the distressing fact was the uncertainty, a thousand thoughts hovering in my mind that ran recklessly. The anticipation was grueling. My husband didn't get to rest much while I was in the ICU for 6 days. It was Navratri time, and my mother fasted all the 9 days with the hope that I will return home healthy with happy news.

Naresh slept outside the ICU and waited the whole night to be allowed entry inside at 4 am in the morning. I too waited desperately to see him in the morning, unable to sleep the whole night. It was the worst feeling, and discomfort didn't let me sleep.

Often relatives visited at home or the hospital. More than comforting me, they taunted me, "We expected to hear some good news from you, but things are quite different here." This made me feel even more disheartened, and I began losing courage. I didn't ever want to be in such a situation again.

They had prescribed a medicine that forced me to urinate continuously. Since I was unable to stand or walk, I needed the bedpan. The nurse got fed up with me; I needed it very frequently. It irritated her, and she lost her patience. She refused to come over when I called for her. Well, there are a lot of side effects of IVF that don't get discussed but in my case, since I faced hyperstimulation, I was majorly affected.

We requested the nurse to help me when I pressed the bell and called her. As she herself was tired, I requested her, "I'm in pain, so please help me. I do understand that I'm disturbing you. But, I can't do much as I'm going through hell. I can't even get up."

We paid her some cash so that she doesn't neglect my call. After 6 days, I was discharged, and my husband decided to take me in a sedan instead of an ambulance.

While going back home, I couldn't rest at all. I was weak and was unable to sit comfortably. I felt like urinating, and we didn't get a place where I could go and urinate. Only my husband was there with me. With not a woman around, I was even more uncomfortable.

Naresh used a bedsheet to cover me so that I could sit and urinate in the pan. Sitting also was a herculean task for me due to immense pain. I was taken on a stretcher and admitted to the hospital in Kalyan since I needed to be observed by the doctor. I needed a stretcher as I could barely stand due to weakness. There was a strike in Bombay Hospital; thus, I got discharged inspite of not having fully recovered. We had to wait for 15 more days for the Beta-hCG test.

I cannot express my feelings about how I felt after returning home. You know, when people go on a long unplanned journey they don't wish to be on, they struggle to return home. When they do, it feels like heaven. A feeling of being in your mother's womb where no one can harm you, a place so safe in the whole world is your home. But unfortunately, I couldn't go to my mother's home. My husband insisted that I should return back to his home. Four more days were left and I would be on the journey to motherhood. I was on top of the world, believing that nothing could stop me.

We all live amidst our people; safe and secure. We can't even imagine how it is to be in a situation where we are helpless. But desires and dreams drive us. They make us move mountains, don't they?

After four days of anxious anticipation, the moment of truth arrived with the Beta-hCG test. With bated breath, we awaited the results, clinging to hope amidst a sea of uncertainty.

But as the test results came back, our worst fears were realized—it was negative. The crushing weight of disappointment bore down on us, leaving us feeling utterly dejected and defeated.

At that moment, it felt as though our dreams had been shattered, our hopes dashed against the harsh reality of our situation.

I had put my body under this torture that it certainly didn't deserve. I mishandled myself and had done grave injustice to it. I needed a break – I needed love, care and affection. It was a Sunday when Naresh suddenly suggested, "Geeta, let's take a break. We have been so busy and preoccupied with treatments, medicines and visits to the hospital. It's a bit too stressful."

Really glad with his suggestion and relieved too I instantly agreed, "Yes, we should go but where? Do you have any plans?"

"Goa, what say?" bang came his reply.

"Done, let's go." I replied excitedly.

We spent a week in Goa relaxing at the beautiful shores, gazing at the sparkling water, sitting for hours hand in hand, enjoying the serene beaches and silence. The best was the Vainguinim Beach with no crowd at all, as compared to other beaches abuzz with people. It was a great place to unwind, away from our busy schedules.

The churches in Goa are so beautiful; the peace and tranquility prevailing in the churches made me introspect about how far we had traveled, consumed by desire and hope. The quietness, stillness, and silence certainly calmed both of us. The day before we left for Mumbai, we visited the churches and carried along with us a settled and stress-free mind.

We never spoke about anything regarding the treatment and our lives in Mumbai, as if we had entered a completely different world; a fairy tale world.

When we came back, things were the same. The routine set in.

I was crawling back to normal yet not giving up on my dream!

Chapter 6

Hope: The Reason to Keep Going

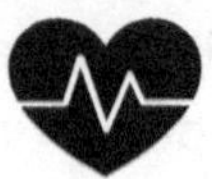

Hope is not delusion, it's the cause of survival and everything beautiful that is existing in this world.

After we were back from Goa, we chose to try IVF one more time at Venkatesh Hospital with reduced dosages for lesser side effects and it failed.

Naresh and I were doing great in business. The sales were boosted by a well-defined strategy, where the counseling part was handled by me and the training part was taken care of by Naresh. The enrollments were high and students were happy since they were getting placed in companies they aimed to be employed.

We both decided to open a Dombivili branch in 2007. Mr. Naik was not too happy about the fact that Pooja was handling the inquiries at Thane branch so we shifted Pooja to the Dombivali branch as a counselor.

But, a new challenge awaited us.

September 15, 2008, Lehman Brothers filed for bankruptcy.

The year 2008 hit the IT market in the most gruesome way. Retrenchments began and Indian companies suffered a major setback. U.S. companies that outsourced projects to Indian IT giants and other companies started withdrawing projects. The global economic recession forced companies to reduce hiring, freeze salaries and postpone new projects. Employees in the IT sectors, like software programmers and call center executives, were laid off.

Indians were losing jobs and our business hit an all-time low. The stock market collapsed. The Lehman Brothers filed for bankruptcy inspite of the fact they were given an investment grade rating by big rating agencies just before they filed for bankruptcy. They lacked the sufficient collateral to borrow from the Federal Reserve. The Lehman Brothers collapsed because a large part of the mortgages they allowed homebuyers were without assessing their capacity to repay the loans. When they defaulted on their loans in large numbers, the entire financial system collapsed.

It's true that greed can destroy everything - families, relationships, and the entire economy too.

We had chosen IVF because we could afford it while our business ran successfully. But now, our business was suffering, and since IVF was not working out for us, we chose to try alternative therapies like homeopathy and Ayurveda.

Homeopathic treatment did not involve much effort except for the initial 2 appointments where a lot of information about my nature, habits, childhood, food habits, daily routine, preferences, our relationship, etc., were probed in great detail. The first appointment went on for around one hour where the doctor covered most aspects of my life.

It was an exhaustive session, but I answered each question with great patience with the hope that this would work for us. I tried this treatment for around 6 months with no conclusive results. My dosages and the kind of medicine were modulated. Our doctor kept on consoling me, but results didn't come our way.

Disappointed and dejected, I started losing heart, and my mood was always morose.

Looking at an energetic person like me slowly slipping into this miserable state of mind, Naresh felt disheartened. Our routine was on, though business was not doing well. That tension was lingering too.

Naresh and I usually returned home together from the office. Now, almost 9 months had passed, and we were so busy in our lives that taking a break was necessary. On the way back home, Naresh handed over an envelope to me.

"What is this now?" I worriedly asked.

"Open it na baby," he lovingly replied.

Disinterested in it, I opened the envelope only to be absolutely thrilled.

"Kashmir, we are going to Kashmir. Seriously. Unbelievable."

The weekend we traveled to Gulmarg, I was convinced Kashmir is heaven.

Like Amir Khusrow said,

"Agar firdaus bar roo-e zameen ast, Hameen ast-o hameen ast-o hameen ast."

If there is a heaven on earth, it's here, it's here…

The scenic beauty of Himalayan mountains in the backdrop of Gulmarg, 'The valley of flowers', looked beautiful, and I carry those memories with me even today. As we took the cable car at Gondola, we could witness nature's delight as we passed the valley. I kept wondering, how could God make such a beautiful place and humans are trying to destroy it through the years for their selfish ends. We also visited Sonamarg, Shalimar Garden, Kupwara.

The terrain of Kashmir is diverse; blessed with dense forest of Kupwara, rich flora of Sonamarg with silver birch, fir, alpine flowers, and saffron plantations at Pampore district of Kashmir valley.

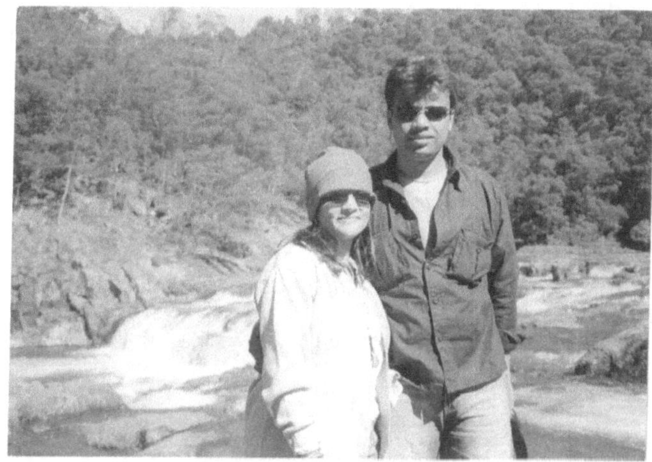

We traveled to Shalimar Bagh which has arched niches along with waterfalls that look like a fairy tale land in the night when the niches are lit up. Our romance bloomed in Kashmir, and we were getting closer. It was a trip that I wished never ended. We were so close and carefree, immersed in each other's arms as if our world began, existed and ended just there.

Not for even a second, we thought about our lives back in Mumbai. Kashmir is a place where souls meet, cherish memories and become inseparable. That is how Kashmir is, 'Unforgettable.'

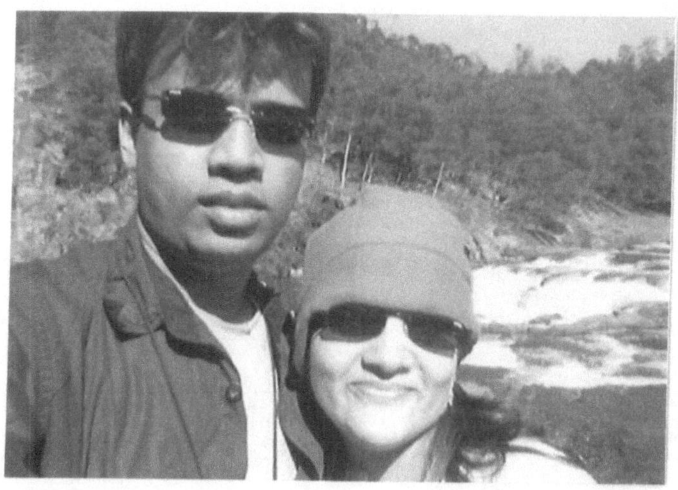

Naresh deeply cared for me, so ensured that even amidst our stress-filled life and ongoing treatments, we took regular breaks to such awesome places. After this memorable trip to Kashmir, we were back, and life had a lot more for us in store, some undiscovered paths, and some more moments of challenges to be faced together.

[1] Ovarian hyperstimulation syndrome (OHSS): When a woman's ovaries are swollen, and they leak fluid into the body. It occurs in cases when women get treated for infertility, and the ovaries are stimulated to boost the production of eggs.

Chapter 7

Back to IVF

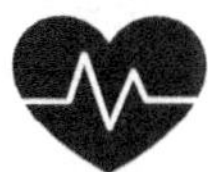

Challenges are a part and parcel of life. No matter how famished, overcoming them makes life beautiful.

We faced a financial crunch, and over and above that, we had invested money in buying our office premises. Naresh began to work as a corporate trainer at Pragati, while I was handling our business. This came as a blessing to us, since he had uploaded his resume on different portals and he received an offer to train Wipro employees. So, he needed to travel Pan India (Hyderabad, Chennai, Mumbai, Bangalore). Our financial challenges started getting resolved, and we both were truly happy. We had waited for a long time for our financial stability to return, and owing to Naresh's new profile, we were back on track.

In 2010, we now felt a bit stable and settled, and the desire of having a child was still on Naresh's mind. We were in 2010, and it had been 5 years of marriage. I hoped that Naresh must have given up on the idea of having a child. Looking at my health, he would suggest opting for adoption. But, no, that wasn't the case.

He was on tour, and I knew he wouldn't be there on my birthday. I had looked at his schedule and knew very well that he wouldn't be able to make it to my birthday. But between trainings in different cities, the company often gave a day's break, and Naresh managed to come home on my birthday and surprise me.

I was extremely happy that he made it to my birthday. But something else was awaiting me, and he seemed to be vividly occupied with something on his mind, of which I was unaware about. Naresh was jubilant and broke the news that worried and tensed me to no extent,

"Now things look financially stable, let's try IVF once again."

I didn't wish to go through the ordeal again. The pain, emotional and physical stress came back in a gush, and I wanted to scream, "No, not again. I cannot take this anymore. Don't, please don't make me go through this trauma again."

Frankly, I didn't wish to disappoint him and simply said, "Okay, dear."

Thus, begins the IVF journey with another doctor. We approached Dr. Feroza Parekh for IVF at Jaslok Hospital this time, and she was known as one of the best doctors. The day we went to the hospital, I was pretty nervous about Dr. Parekh's response and diagnosis. She advised us some more tests and concluded that I had Tuberculosis in my uterus that prevented me from conceiving. The endometrial lining in the uterus was thick and hindered the implantation of the fetus.

We felt so disappointed because if Dr. Venkatesh had diagnosed this, I wouldn't have had to go through so much pain, and I would have conceived by now.

Dr. Parekh said, "We cannot go for IVF now. I advise you to take a treatment for 9 months to cure Tuberculosis." Though I was happy that I got a break from IVF and that we needed to wait for 9 more months before the IVF journey restarted, but every month I needed to go for a monthly check-up at Jaslok Hospital.

There used to be a long line where I needed to stand to get my uterus lining checked through a sonography. People from around the world consulted her, so it used to be pretty crowded there. So when I traveled to Jaslok Hospital to get the uterus lining checked, my sisters and mother waited patiently for the latest report. I had also begun having ghee sourced from the famous Ayurvedic and yoga Guru Ramdev Baba, which I mixed in milk and drank every morning. This improved the lining and ultimately after 8 to 9 months, the lining had improved, and we could go ahead with IVF.

The same process was repeated, and the routine began. The embryo was transferred, and I had already informed the doctor that I'm prone to hyperstimulation. They took enough care while transferring the embryo. Inspite of it, I was in discomfort. So, I was admitted to the hospital, and my stomach started swelling, and as earlier, I was unable to pass urine. They kept me under observation at the hospital for 15 days till Beta-hCG results would be out.

Naresh was by my side for 15 days and didn't go home at all. The doctors advised him to go home since I was just under observation, but he refused to go home to focus on business. My health and having a baby was his top priority, and he didn't want to take any chances. He knew one thing, "We have come here together and we shall leave together." This support meant a lot to me.

Ultimately, the day dawned when the Beta-hCG would be done. Even today, as those memories flashback, I feel nervous. I was watching TV in my room and heard the astrological predictions for my zodiac sign, Scorpio, and it wasn't too positive, which made me nervous. I immediately switched off the TV and desperately waited for the results.

I still remember the date; it was 30th June 2012. Naresh was by my side awaiting the doctor's response, and at that moment, nothing else seemed to be important in this world. Having a child was our biggest dream, and this report made us nervous.

We waited to be called into Dr. Feroza Parekh's cabin. We couldn't even wait for a second more, and the wait was unbearable.

"You can go inside," said the receptionist.

We looked at each other, and both of us were tensed.

"Why do you both look so tensed? We have good news, the report is positive."

I literally fell at the doctor's feet and thanked her. For me, she was a Goddess who had blessed me with a child.

I was ready to face any pain or discomfort since my dream was soon going to come true.

God had been kind to us, so our business was flourishing. In my absence, Pooja looked after both Kalyan and Dombivali branches single-handedly. We were at peace since we knew someone from our own family was running the show at both the branches. Pooja was trained for some other reason, but now her work came in handy to us while I was away. Nature supports us when our resolve is strong.

I was jubilant, but the discomfort hadn't gone away. My stomach was bulging, and it was stiff. The next morning at 4 p.m., I had severe pain. The doctor advised me to walk to mobilize the water accumulated in my stomach.

While I was walking in the hospital, people looking at the bulge on my stomach began asking me, "Is it the 7th or the 8th month?" This made me even more nervous. When the pain became unbearable and the bulge didn't recede, my husband reached out to the doctor. They immediately punctured my stomach on the right-hand side and removed the excess water accumulated. Since I was pregnant, they had to be extra careful, and we all were worried that the baby shouldn't be harmed. Ultimately, after puncturing my stomach and removing the excess water content, I could relax and go to sleep. I was in the hospital for a few more days and then discharged. I hated the hospital food, so my mother sent homemade food from Ulhasnagar. We weren't allowed to bring homemade food into the hospital, but we somehow smuggled it.

We had ultimately realized our dream; I was carrying our baby - the most awaited moment of my life was here. Tears flowed down my cheeks; I held Naresh tight and cried like a baby. My happiness knew no bounds - after such a long wait, I would ultimately be a mother, and the tiny toddler would fill our lives with laughter and happiness.

I went back home, and my mother-in-law showered all her love on me. She performed the ritual to remove all the bad omens that could have attracted to me (it is called as 'nazar utarna'). But I missed the food cooked by my mother, though I didn't go to live with her as I wanted to spend time with Naresh.

They pampered me and took a lot of care. The affection and pampering that I had longed for had come my way. Things weren't as simple as they might seemed. We had to travel all the way to Breach Candy near Jaslok Hospital every month for a sonography and various tests to ensure the good health of the baby. There is a test called the **Triple Screen Test (or Triple Marker), where birth defects can be determined. That too was normal by God's grace.**

Day by day, things started progressing, and we were super excited that soon I would be giving birth to a baby and our house would be filled with the sweet sounds of a baby.

I loved the baby bump and was super excited feeling my baby by stroking my abdomen. I loved talking to my baby and felt her move. Well, she was a baby girl; I was extremely sure about it. I chatted with her and told her how special she was, that I awaited her eagerly. Hitting a conversation with my child was probably the first step to motherhood. I didn't know what was in store for me.

Now I was consulting a gynecologist, Dr. Anahita, at Jaslok Hospital who advised me in the fourth month to keep consulting a local gynecologist as well. But we were too anxious and didn't wish to take the risk of consulting some other doctor, so we decided that the delivery should be done at Jaslok Hospital itself. We had begun preparing for the Godh Bharai function held in the seventh month.

I was at home away from the office and my daily routine, feeling left out. But I explained to myself that it's okay because having a baby was my innate desire that was getting fulfilled so I could sacrifice anything for this dream. I began looking different due to a lot of hair loss and acne on my face. In fact, I lost weight as well and looked weak. But these things were secondary too.

Everyone had already begun to celebrate, and it was an occasion everyone had been waiting for a long time. As the day was nearing, we all were so happy. Having a baby was our dream for a long time, and we had seen tough times together. The baby would bring new energy into our lives and a joy that was incomparable to anything else in the world.

While we were all rejoicing and the house was filled with positive vibes, one day when I woke up and had a bath after performing my daily puja, I felt heavy. This was a weird and uncomfortable feeling. It felt as if I was getting periods. I feared bleeding and frequently visited the washroom to check and ensure everything was normal.

The next day, the discomfort became even more severe. I felt a pinch in my stomach as if it was getting pulled and then released. This feeling continued for some time. I was totally unaware that this was labor pain that I was experiencing. I bore the pain till afternoon, but then the pain aggravated. I still remember we had a ceremony (Mata ki chowki) at our home. My cousin came to pick me up to travel to my mother's home. I shared with him about the discomfort and pain. So, he immediately took me to the doctor, and my husband traveled from the Kalyan office to the doctor's clinic as well. But I couldn't even manage to stand in the lift or sit, so I just slept at the table in the waiting room.

I kept anxiously asking my husband, "I hope we will be able to save our child."

Naresh kept comforting me, "Don't worry, Geeta, you and the baby both will be fine. Just try to relax yourself."

After some time, the doctor came to his cabin, and we were called inside. As I was lying on the bench, with great effort, I picked myself up with the help of Naresh and got up. The doctor checked me only to say,

"This is a case of IVF, and I cannot advise. You need to go back to the consulting doctor. Take her to Jaslok Hospital in the ambulance at the earliest."

Naresh immediately called Dr. Anahita, who fired the local doctor, "Geeta is in pain; you cannot make her travel to Jaslok Hospital. It's too far. I hope you understand the emergency; it's not safe for her to travel."

It was evident that my pain was unbearable and it was getting severe. A lot of time was wasted in this communication. The doctor concluded that they needed to stitch the vagina since it was just the fifth month. They made preparations in the operation theater, and I was lying on the bed when the nurse was about to cleanse the vagina to begin stitching it and the water spluttered on her face like a fountain, and the fetus got pushed out completely.

This was the ultimate disaster, and we were obviously shocked. I couldn't see the baby or rather was not allowed to see my child. The ones who saw mentioned that she was tall, just like my husband. The doctors tried to save her life by incubating, but she was too young and this facility was not available here in India. She was finally buried, and I never saw my beautiful child. The connection I had developed while the tiny life within me stayed for 5 months broke in just a few minutes. I couldn't bear this trauma and felt like ending my life.

Innumerable times I felt like committing suicide. How could nature be so cruel to me while I was trying so hard to give birth to a child that it refused to oblige? My entire team, family, and relatives were at the hospital. They were so shocked and didn't know how to console me. I was crying and was uncontrollable.

When the nurse was injecting me to stop lactation, I got totally shattered. I cried endlessly as my dream of feeding my baby was shattered. When I was discharged after 3 days and came back home, life became meaningless. I was traumatized and got up screaming each night.

Now things completely changed for me, Naresh, and his family.

Chapter 8
The Conflict

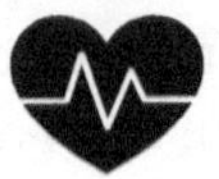

**Prolonged silence can hurt. Silence is not always
the remedy to hurt and pain.**

Everyone was upset and stressed at Naresh's home, but they hid it from us. They never revealed their true feelings and tried to keep the environment at home very light and cordial. A lot of the credit goes to my mother-in-law, who shielded us from all the questions, sympathy, and unnecessary conversations from everyone. She wouldn't let anyone say a word to me and Naresh. She was my greatest support system, and that is why I respect her the most.

But no one quit the idea of having a baby. In fact, they said it is possible to have a baby since it happened once; we could see success in the future. They tried to console me or probably themselves, so I felt a bit tense that even after such a tedious and tiring journey, we failed miserably yet no one was ready to think from my point of view. I was emotionally and mentally exhausted.

My mother-in-law ensured that she took good care of me and did everything she could. The post-pregnancy care that was necessary was given to me along with a 40-day massage routine and healthy food cooked by her. Despite the fact that I didn't have my baby with me, I had to undergo a post-pregnancy routine and care. The lady who came over for a massage encouraged me by explaining that this is necessary for your future pregnancies. What an irony! I didn't have a baby, but I had to undergo post-pregnancy care. This hurt me to no extent, and I had begun sulking.

Often, I thought over and engaged in a monologue, "Geeta, giving birth to a child is so important for you? Look at you!! You've tried everything in the world; tortured your body, mind, and soul. What more do you wish to do?"

The answer was simple, "I wish Naresh and his family to be happy. And they will be happy only when they see our baby. The wish of being grandparents was very much alive in his parents' hearts."

Instead of sulking at home, going to the office was a better option. So, I convinced my mother-in-law that I needed to divert my mind by going to the office, and she understood my point of view. But her only condition was that I should complete the 40 days massage and eat all the nutritious food cooked by her. She herself cooked various nutritious dishes for me, which most Maharashtrian women are given during post-pregnancy care. She was preparing my body for future pregnancies. I felt deeply hurt and disappointed; despite the harsh fact that I couldn't give them a child, she did everything for me.

My periods were still irregular, and that disappointed me to no extent. After a few days passed when I felt a bit relaxed, we reapproached Dr. Feroza Parekh for a follow-up. This time they gave a new reason for my not being able to conceive.

I still remember the day we entered the same hospital premises again. I was nervous; mentally and emotionally, I wasn't strong enough to undergo another round of IVF. Outside her consulting room, I kept looking at the faces of to-be mothers. Some looked happy, some nervous, while others looked vividly tired. Being a mother is the biggest gift nature has given a woman, and men are bereft of this joy.

"Geeta Khandare, you can go inside. Doctor is calling you," said the receptionist.

I felt heavy and nervous; my stomach began to grumble.

Dr. Feroza looked at me and whispered, "Hello, Geeta. How are you doing now?"

I simply smiled and said, "I'm much better."

"Fine, we need to go for some more tests so that we don't face any issues again," said Dr. Feroza.

We went for the prescribed test, and it was time for Dr. Feroza to guide us and tell us the future course of action. I kept praying that everything should be alright.

Sitting in front of her while she checked the report felt like an unending wait; I eagerly awaited her opinion that came, and it was not too positive.

She said, "You are not able to conceive because you have excess AOA (Anti-Ovarian Antibodies), which doesn't let a foreign body stay within the body, and the sperm injected from outside is a foreign body too."

My shoulders and my entire body sunk in the chair. I felt helpless. This time there was a new reason as a barrier to my motherhood.

I doubted the credibility of the doctor and was so furious that she was completely oblivious to the pain and trauma I had gone through. Was it all so simple for them? Why couldn't they diagnose the challenges the first time itself? Do I have to go through the same trauma again and again?

"Why me?" I screamed from within. I just wish this scream reaches the Almighty, and he brings me out of this vicious cycle.

Naresh looked at me and held my hand to ask the doctor, "What do you advise us to do now?"

Dr. Feroza said, "We need to give her drips that control AOA in her body."

I was always confident about Dr. Feroza, so I continued consulting her. I didn't have the guts to ask her, "Why wasn't this diagnosed earlier and cured?"

Physically, mentally, emotionally, and financially, we were completely drained. But there was no point in arguing. Every month we visited the hospital for the drip. Meanwhile, I consulted my friend who is a doctor and resides in Germany. She confirmed that AOA doesn't allow women to conceive, and the treatment is accurate.

Every month we traveled from Kalyan to Jaslok Hospital, for the procedure (drip) of controlling AOA. The wait was long, and I was slowly losing patience. Post this course of drip given to me completed, we tried IVF again. They had a few of our frozen embryos and tried injecting them, but all the attempts failed miserably.

During these tough times, my journey to live a healthy life began.

Chapter 9
Healthy and Happy Life

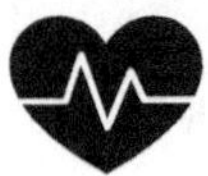

Your body is the vehicle on which dreams are driven.

Living a healthy life is a choice you make.

Naresh asked me once,

"Why don't you join gym?"

I plainly replied, "How will that change things?"

Naresh jumped in excitement, "Just at least begin coming to the gym; you will know how it feels. When you lose a few pounds and look at yourself in the mirror all slim and trim, I bet it will excite you. The way you look at yourself will change completely. Aao toh sahi."

Naresh had been gyming for more than a decade and is a fitness freak. I was never so particular about my health and had put on a lot of weight after marriage.

All that I thought was let me try once and see how it actually feels since Naresh was so excited to have me there.

With a lot of resistance, I began visiting the gym, and it was a big torture. Sweating it out and burning calories was not an easy task. For almost a month, it was a herculean task to continue gyming. I hated the exercises as they caused muscle ache. For a person like me who had never worked out, gyming was the most hated activity of the day. I felt the jitters about going to the gym.

But I continued, and after a month later, my friend complimented, "You've lost a bit of weight. Looking good yaar!!"

Now my clothes were a bit loose, and I had lost a few inches.

I looked at myself in the mirror and said, "Geeta, just imagine, if you lose more weight, you will look just fab. Wear the clothes you wish and get back in shape."

I had tried walking and yoga. But losing weight had become elusive. I had tried walking 5 km daily. I also practiced yoga and managed to do all asanas.

From the simple Padmasana to Surya Namaskar to the balancing Tadasan. I managed to do all of them. But never lost weight. With gyming, it was a visible change in me that I got addicted to. I was also worried about the PCOD problem that I had, and yoga could resolve that issue. That is what I had heard from people and read as well. That is the reason I joined yoga, but eventually it could not be resolved. Not the weight issue nor my PCOD challenge.

Two months down the line after gyming, I got used to the routine. I did not have a personal coach in the beginning, but eventually Naresh suggested I should have one.

That changed everything about my exercise schedule and routine. He suggested to me what exercises I should be choosing and divided the days into weight training, cardio, and cross-function.

He kept a tab on my exercise schedule and watched how I'm progressing to moderate the exercise routine. Surprisingly, after 3 months, my periods became regular, and this motivated me to continue gymming. Bunking my gym due to any reason was frustrating for me. Missing my exercise routine made me feel I'm stepping backward in my journey toward motherhood. I was surprised that even walking regularly 5 km each day and then trying yoga hadn't helped me in having regular periods.

While life was changing and I experienced weight loss, an amazing book fell into my hands, which also mentioned the benefits of exercising.

I call this miraculous. If you wish for something real bad, everything around you will lead you there. Your strong desire and unfading will is the source of your positive energy.

This book is penned by Nutritionist Rujuta Diwekar called, 'Don't lose your mind.' Lose your weight.'

So, I began observing my eating pattern and my lifestyle once I read this book.

Let me put the insights and tips that she shares in the book. The ones I followed as I was so inspired by her book.

What inspired me?

It's important to change your lifestyle to be able to lose weight. Diet with a primary aim of weight loss is meant to fail.

What changed?

I began working out regularly:

While I felt pathetically bored of exercises and felt that eating properly will help me lose weight, I read her funda, that any weight loss program that doesn't stress on exercise is worthless.

I began working out regularly for an hour each day and became a regular at the gym.

Juices got replaced with whole fruits as she says juices remove minerals and vitamins from them.

- **Quit thinking of going on a strict diet:**

   There was a time when I was thinking of going on a strict diet. But surprisingly, Rujuta discourages doing something like that. Dieting is not starving, she says.

   So, if you want a toned and muscular body, you have to respect your stomach and love it. Why load your stomach with something it cannot digest?

- **Became observant:**

   I began observing what I eat and when I eat. I realized that I was practicing an incorrect lifestyle, which stopped me from losing weight.

Often when I got bored, as a distraction, I ate some chocolates, consoling myself that it's good once in a while. But the craving did not become less - it built up. So I reached for more food, and this too is mentioned in her book.

- **Eat 2 hours before you sleep:**

I had a late dinner and that too a heavy one. While she says we need to have a light dinner as the digestive system works slowly at night. We also need to have food 2 hours before sleeping as it aids digestion.

- **Understood the myth about overeating:**

Through the years, I also ate more than I was capable of digesting. This was my issue. But I needed to be aware that I was doing that. If the stomach lacks the fire to digest at a given time, then even a bit of food is overeating. So, eating food at the wrong time is overeating. Not just eating large quantities of food is overeating. I realized that every time I take an extra bit of food, even if I know I'm done with my meal, it means I'm overfeeding myself.

- **Stop storing sweets in the freezer:**

Also, our freezer used to be stored with sweets, ice-cream, and mithai due to festivals. We stopped doing that as it became a habit to gorge on sweets and fried foods.

I also began eating every 2 hours, bit by bit, and that too mindfully as she says.

It's true that I became more attentive about what my stomach was saying to me and its need for food.

- **Quit watching TV, switched off my phone and computer while having food:**

Also, I quit watching TV while having food as she mentions that you have to involve all your senses while having food.

Rightly put by Dr. Divekar, we have to watch what we eat instead of watching television; we have to watch our food. All our senses should be involved while we have our food so that we don't overeat and listen to our stomach signaling that we ate enough.

Also, I switch off my phone and computer.

- **Avoid refrigerated food:**

I began to avoid keeping food in the freezer and consumed it within 3 hours of cooking.

I quit drinking tea as soon as I got up. Made it a habit to have real food within 10 to 15 minutes after waking up. When we get up, our state of mind is relaxed and so is our body.

- **I also started eating my last meal 2 hours before sleeping.**

Also, she says good quality, restful, and peaceful sleep is the backbone of losing fat.

When you sleep, the body rejuvenates and repairs. If you eat 2 hours before going to bed, most of the food gets digested before you go to bed, you get a sound sleep, your body is all ready to do the repairing, and this helps burn fat.

Insight:

- I loved the fact she put in her book that the human body is meant for continuous activity.

- Also, there is nothing like 'safe food' or 'fattening food.' Eating at the right time and in the right quantity is important.

- She says that once we have a calmer mind, we are ready to break down the food to digest it. And that way food reaches deep inside us, to all tissue. This needs energy. Stress actually adds fat.

- Carbs help to burn fat so you need carbs, so don't remove them completely from your diet. In the absence of carbs, fat cannot be utilized for energy.

- Honey, lime water/apple cider vinegar. These are magical drinks that I believed and was told by others. But she says it's a myth and can actually work against you. Do buy the book and read to understand how she explains the reason.

- Stress makes the digestive system sluggish. A relaxed body and mind are good for your health and avoid adding fat.

- Eating every 2 hours:

  ➤ It helps to burn fat.

  ➤ Few calories are converted to fat.

  ➤ Brain gets a regular flow of sugar so you think smarter.

  ➤ Flatter stomach.

- Also, if you are less active, eat less and eat more when you are more active. When you eat every 2 hours, the meal size decreases when you are less active. When you follow these principles, you are in touch with your hunger signals and listen to them.

- I asked myself, "Do I really care about what my stomach needs?" The answer was 'no.' I usually just kept loading it according to my convenience.

While I was involved in living a healthy life, I got the news that my sister Bharati had conceived through IVF. Surprisingly, the IVF procedure suited Bharati who lived in Dubai. She also suffered from PCOD. Bharati had approached Dr. Feroza Parekh due to my recommendation as I truly believed she was a great doctor. Bharati had visited India and completed the process of transferring the embryo post which she traveled back to Dubai, while I couldn't even move. She felt no pain at all in the entire process. Her Beta-hCG report was conducted in Dubai before mine and it was positive. This added the hope that my report can be positive too since I was not in much pain this time nor did I have any symptoms of hyperstimulation.

I asked her to send her reports to me, and I derived the conclusion that she had twins since I had become a pro at reading these reports. The doctor confirmed too that she had twins. You would be surprised to know that only 2 embryos got created in Bharati's case, while in my case many embryos were created. Though she started bleeding in the third month and she lost one baby.

My sisters stood by me, but Naresh had stopped talking to me. When I stayed with my mother for a few days after the miscarriage, he hardly came over.

With so many failures, he was exasperated due to this never-ending ordeal. He failed to make sense of this situation. I had let out my emotions by crying, but his emotions had bottled up. He hadn't expressed his pain to anyone openly. Though after my miscarriage, he had hugged my brother-in-law and wept a lot. He hid his dismay, pain, and deluge of emotions, but from within he was broken, and it only transpired to silence. All our efforts to feel the love of a child were rejected by nature, downright cruel, brutal, and savage.

Now they told us that we wouldn't go for the frozen embryos, we should go for a fresh cycle. It was in 2015 that was the last IVF cycle we chose to go for because if this one failed, I had decided to go for surrogacy.

I would save a good amount of money for surrogacy and go for it. If nature was not cooperating with the IVF process inspite of the quality of sperms and eggs being superior, this could be the only way out.

Jaslok Hospital had a program and a department where they would arrange for the surrogate and take care of the pregnancy, which would cost Rs. 25 lakhs back then. But if we arrange for a surrogate, the cost would be just Rs. 5 lakhs. So, I began desperately searching for a surrogate.

Financially, I had stabilized since I had moved to launching a business of corporate training with my brother-in-law, Melwyn. I was doing well in business with him. I had quit our original business and moved ahead with corporate trainings. That was the most challenging period for our marriage. Naresh got very upset and we argued to no extent till the point of opting for divorce.

Since we weren't working together anymore as I had quit business, so the time I spent with Naresh was least. Our dream of having a happy family with kids had collapsed. Nothing was really working out for us. Professionally I was growing but my personal life went for a toss.

Our relationship was not flourishing. We had drifted apart since my profile demanded me to stay connected with decision-makers in various companies, which kept me very busy. My communication was now minimal with Naresh. I enjoyed the profile since it provided me with the satisfaction that was rare in the retail field. My paychecks were high and they came on time. This gave me a kick and I simply loved it.

Initially, my brother-in-law and I operated from Kalyan but since he insisted on having an office we shifted to Thane.

But I still had not given up on the idea of having a baby. I kept watching the videos that showed how the egg and sperm meet to give birth to an embryo. All that I said to myself was,

"This looks so simple, but this could never happen to me. I'm bereft of this simple natural biological process in my life. Giving birth is natural but not in my case."

Chapter 10:
Know Thyself

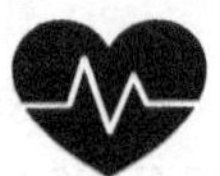

Stay connected to your body, mind, and soul.

While I put efforts into improving my lifestyle and health, I kept thinking, "How can I make Naresh happy? He is the driving force of my life, and I couldn't see him so unhappy."

His face began looking fierce, and he kept gazing emptily as he stood in the balcony for hours. All the pain that had assimilated within him took the form of fierceness. His silence was killing me. So, I decided to speak to my mother-in-law.

The next day, I took a half-day and stayed at home. I approached my mother-in-law and sat down to talk to her.

"Aai, I can clearly see that I cannot keep your son happy. He looks so dissatisfied, and we are constantly fighting. After trying so many times, we didn't have a baby. You should get him married to someone else. At least let him be happy."

She looked straight into my eyes and replied, "This is the first and last time you've said this. You are not supposed to say this again. Have I made myself clear? We will go and perform a Pooja at Udipi, Subramanya, and then our Kuldevi.

After which, we begin with a new treatment at Balaji Tambe." I was happy about spending time with Naresh on this trip.

As planned, we went to Subramanya Temple in Udipi, Mangalore. We also performed the Kaal Sarpa Dosh Nivaran Pooja to ward off all the bad forces impacting our life.

It was a reassurance that my in-laws truly loved me like their child and they were hopeful.

For the first time in so many years, I wholeheartedly prayed to our Kuldevi and begged her to grant our wish to have a child in the family. I was helpless, and I began crying in front of the deity. I told her that every remedy has been tried till date but I'm not blessed with a child. Now it is in her hands to grant my wish.

But the visit brought back my hope and I felt extremely relaxed.

While returning back home, the fear of beginning with the Balaji Tambe Ayurvedic Panchakarma treatment lingered in my mind as suggested by my friend's aunt and everyone agreed to it.

Me and Naresh went to the center at Lonavala where the rules were extremely strict and the diet was tough to follow too. My mother-in-law packed a lot of homemade food so that before we entered the center we could have some homemade food. But once we reached there, the team asked us to surrender all the food we had carried. The treatment was completely different and the food was cooked in a unique way and we were not used to that kind of food. They gave us ghee to drink and gaumutra too.

We then checked into our rooms and were told that we would have to get up early in the morning for meditation and yoga. Also, a small chit would be given post breakfast about the various treatments we would undergo that day along with the time and venue mentioned on it. The same day treatment began but some more tougher challenges awaited us. The next day when we went for breakfast, there wasn't any proper food served as such. We were served laya that could be dipped in tea or milk. Lunch was a full meal and for dinner only soup was served. Thus, practically the whole day, we consumed food only once. We were not mentally prepared for this kind of a diet.

We underwent different types of treatments.

Svedan:

The treatment began with Svedan, which involved application of special oil over the body followed by a steam bath. In this treatment, toxins get released from our cells, which helps in relaxing the muscles and the entire body.

Antarsnehan:

It included drinking medicated ghee, which would get absorbed throughout the body thus, removing the toxins leading to elasticity of the body.

Virechan:

Erandel tel or Castor Oil was given to drink and it led to loose motions. This treatment was called Virechan, which focused on clearing the gastrointestinal tract and bowels or a kind of detoxification of our system.

Netrabasti:

This is the treatment to help improve eyesight.

Nasya:

Nasya involved a head, shoulder, and neck massage. After this medicine is administered through the nose. So, any issue with sinus, disturbed memory or brain problems are treated through Nasya.

Shirodhara

A steady stream of warm oil is poured gently over the forehead leading to deep relaxation.

The treatments were intense and I started having blackouts.

Frequently visiting the loo to pass stools after consuming Castor Oil made me feel extremely weak.

I had to visit the loo 21 times and among all the people who were admitted we had a competition to see who had to visit the loo the most. Probably that was our way of combating the adversity with some humor and play. We consulted the doctor there as I was feeling extremely exhausted and totally famished.

The doctor there shared,

"Geeta this is similar to a surgery that you have undergone. This is an internal cleansing thus, weakness is a result of this treatment."

My husband's treatment lasted for 15 days, he had to leave. After Naresh left I got totally demotivated.

I quit having the soup in the evening and I waited desperately for my treatment to get over so that I could return back home. Ultimately, my treatment was completed and the doctor explained that this diet had to be followed even after going back home until I conceive. We had to avoid non-vegetarian and spicy food. I was firm about following this diet. I bought laya with the intention that I would maintain the same diet. Weakness post-treatment didn't deter me from continuing this diet as I was determined to have a child.

Ultimately it was time to return home and Naresh came to pick me up, the doctor guided both of us and informed us that I would have to visit the center for 5 days to undergo a treatment called Basti. I was in no frame of mind to undergo one more treatment, so, halfheartedly I said 'yes' and left the center.

After returning home I could see some changes in the house as my in-laws had consulted a Vastu expert. Some crystal balls were kept in the kitchen and my room.

Returning back to my routine was not that easy. I used to travel to Thane and generally visited the gym in the evening. But the doctors at Balaji Tambe Center advised me not to visit the gym in the evening as our body gets into the rest mode and we should not disturb this cycle thus, I began visiting the gym in the mornings.

While following my routine I tried coping up with the same diet followed at the center. After a week of doing so, I shared my challenge with my mother-in-law.

"Aai I cannot follow this diet anymore. What should I do? You suggest a way out."

She understood my challenge,

"Geeta stop this diet and continue eating your normal food. I can understand that you are working the whole day and this food makes you feel weak."

Days passed by and I had it in the back of my mind that I had to return to the center for the Basti treatment, which involved giving an enema of medicated oil and decoction of herbs to clean the colon and maintain the muscle tone. Frankly, I didn't want to go back to the center as I dreaded the treatment so I kept postponing it.

Then, I received a call from the center that 5 days of treatment is pending. I was nervous as I didn't want to go back and the rooms were isolated so I was pretty scared to go alone. Naresh understood that I was avoiding.

"You are not going to the center and spending all your time being busy in business. Why are you not completing this 5 day treatment? What are your priorities, Geeta?" Naresh complained and he stopped talking to me.

But how could I tell him that I hated being at the center due to the diet restrictions. But then I didn't have a choice. I called up my friend Seema Jadhav whose treatment was pending so that we could go together. Seema also wasn't able to conceive. She couldn't afford to pay for an airconditioned room so I decided to stay at the center in a non-ac room with her as I couldn't bear thinking of being alone in the room all by myself. I needed someone.

I called the center before leaving in a car, "We are leaving to come to the center, just wished to inform you."

The doctor there asked me, "When did you last get the periods?"

"Three months back." I replied.

"Get the pregnancy kit and check if you are pregnant." the doctor answered.

"No, that is not needed. Since I have PCOD I often miss my periods. So mention that in the records. Im leaving now." I simply replied with not much seriousness.

She tried explaining to me, "Geeta, we cannot admit you at the center until we ensure that you are not pregnant. We cannot give Basti without this report."

I reluctantly went down to get the kit.

Convinced that it would confirm what I already knew: another negative result. Yet, as I glanced down, my certainty shattered into a million pieces. There, on the test, were two distinct lines. My heart stopped, my mind reeling in disbelief. How could this be? I had steeled myself for disappointment, but this was beyond comprehension.

And then, like a thunderclap in a silent room, the word "pregnant" echoed in my ears. Tears welled up in my eyes, but a smile tinged with disbelief and wonder crept onto my lips. It was a moment of contradiction, a collision of emotions so profound that I could scarcely comprehend them. In that instant, the world seemed to stand still as I grappled with the overwhelming reality of what lay before me.

Naresh was not too happy with me those days. Despite my apprehension, I mustered the courage to call him and share the test result. His response was unexpectedly calm; he suggested we repeat the test. To my disbelief, the second test confirmed the same result: positive. It was as if the ground beneath me had shifted, leaving me grappling with the weight of this newfound reality.

In a whirlwind of emotions, I reached out to my friend to cancel our plans. There was no way I could accompany her now. With a sense of urgency, I made my way to the clinic for a Beta-hCG test, desperate for confirmation. And there it was, staring back at me from the test results: undeniable proof that I was pregnant.

The timing seemed almost surreal—it was Sankashti, a day traditionally associated with auspicious beginnings. Yet, here I was, already three months into a journey I had never expected to embark upon. As I processed the news, a wave of conflicting emotions washed over me, leaving me simultaneously terrified and inexplicably hopeful for what lay ahead. Then I could relate the reasons behind the blackouts and weakness. I thanked God for saving my child through the intense treatment in the initial months of pregnancy. Though I was fully drained out mentally and physically, my child was safe and it was not less than a miracle.

The journey toward living a holistic healthy life began a year and a half back. While I was still contemplating the reasons that led to my pregnancy, I realized it's my changed lifestyle that had been a blessing in disguise.

Unknowingly I had walked on a path that led me to the fulfillment of my dream. I waited for so long and completely relied on unnatural methods.

We are generally so impatient in our lives; we never listen to the signals our body keeps on indicating but we just ignore them as we are so busy in our daily routine. Often we lack faith in ourselves and God as well. We rely too much on people's comments and doctors' opinions completely. Do we ever pause for a moment and sit peacefully to feel our breath, the subtle sound of our breath and what our mind says?

In July 2016, when I was already 3 months pregnant, I resigned from the venture that I had collaborated with my brother-in-law. I stayed at home for 6 months taking rest. Though I felt really sad since going to meet my sister Bharati, after she delivered was impossible. My lifestyle was stress-free with no work at all and I focused on reading a lot for those 9 months.

People often talk about pregnancy but never talk about miscarriage. Now, every time I went for an ultrasound I felt nervous; it was like giving an exam totally possessed by the fear of failing. I felt confused whether I should be nervous or celebrate but, eventually, I learned to trust my body.

Though I was pretty tense and didn't want to go through the agony of miscarriage, so I frequently visited the bathroom to ensure there was no spotting. Overall, the mood at home was happy, and my mother-in-law was so happy upon hearing the news that I was expecting that she cooked Dal Pakwan (a Sindhi delicacy). Life had changed and we went for morning walks regularly as it could aid natural delivery.

Despite the joyous atmosphere surrounding us, there was a tinge of sadness as December approached. My beloved brother Tarun was about to embark on a new chapter of his life, stepping into marriage, a momentous occasion that I had long looked forward to celebrating alongside him. However, with my pregnancy now in its eighth month, attending his wedding seemed like an impossible dream.

But amidst the sorrow, I knew that my absence should not cast a shadow over his special day. With a heavy heart, I mustered the courage to make a difficult decision. I urged Naresh and our family to attend the wedding, ensuring that my brother wouldn't feel the sting of my absence.

In a heartwarming display of solidarity, my dear friend Sheetal facilitated a video call, allowing me to witness the ceremony from afar. Though separated by distance, our spirits remained connected, bridging the gap between us in a moment of shared love and celebration.

As I watched my brother exchange vows with his beloved, tears welled up in my eyes. His emotions were palpable even through the screen, his heart heavy with the absence of his cherished sister. It was a bittersweet moment, a testament to the bond that bound us together, even in moments of separation.

Though I longed to be by his side, dancing and celebrating in person, my priority lay elsewhere. With each kick and flutter from within, my baby reminded me of the precious new life growing inside me, a life that demanded my undivided attention and care.

In January, my mother-in-law arranged godbharia (Indian baby shower).

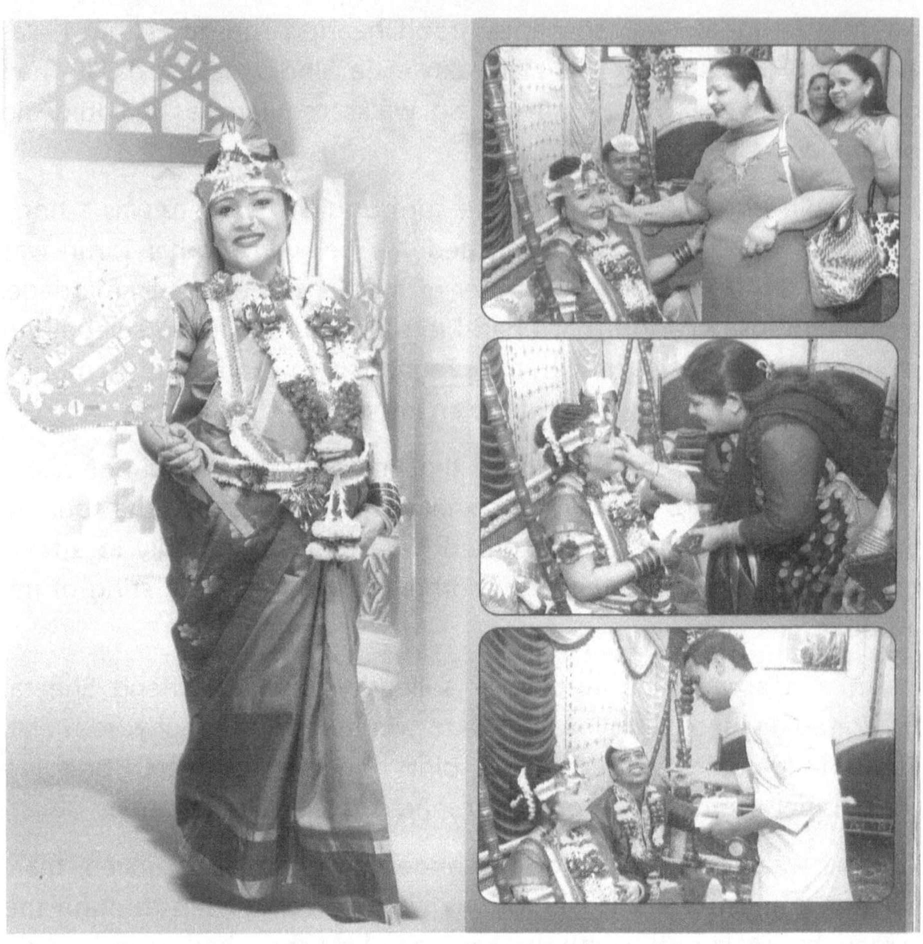

There were around 200 people who attended the function though I was a bit reluctant to celebrate at this point of time. All I wanted was a safe delivery.

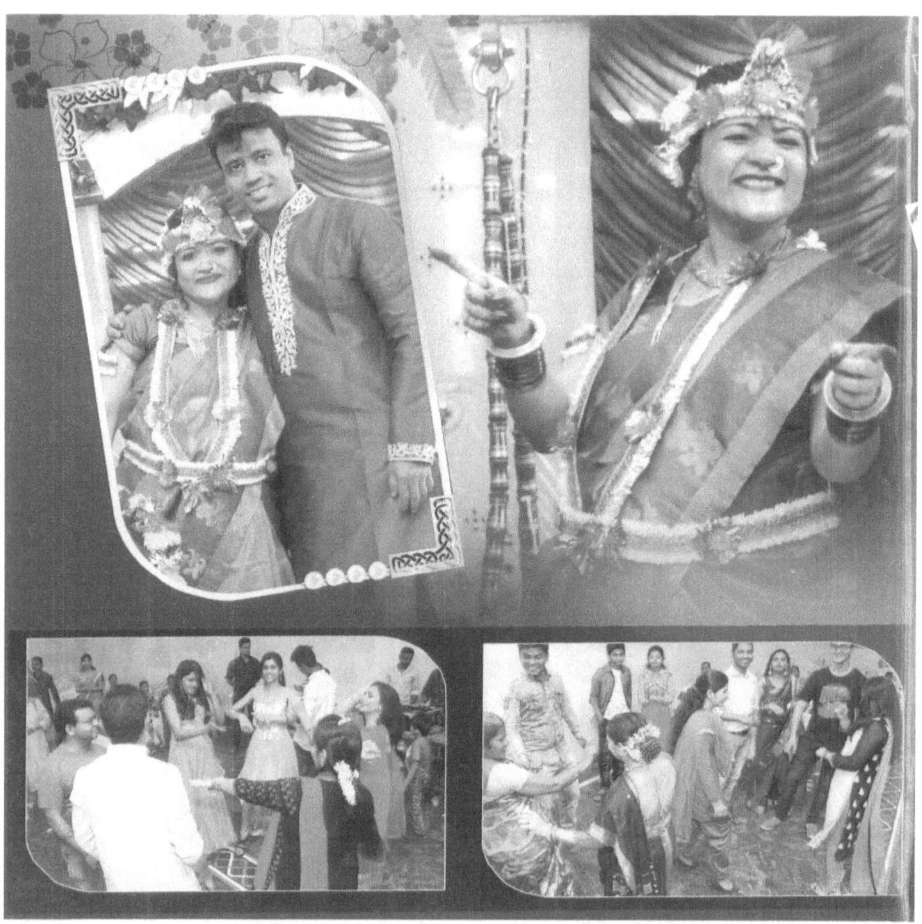

In fact, relatives and friends who attended the baby shower were more as compared to my marriage ceremony. It was a memorable celebration and we all were jubilant.

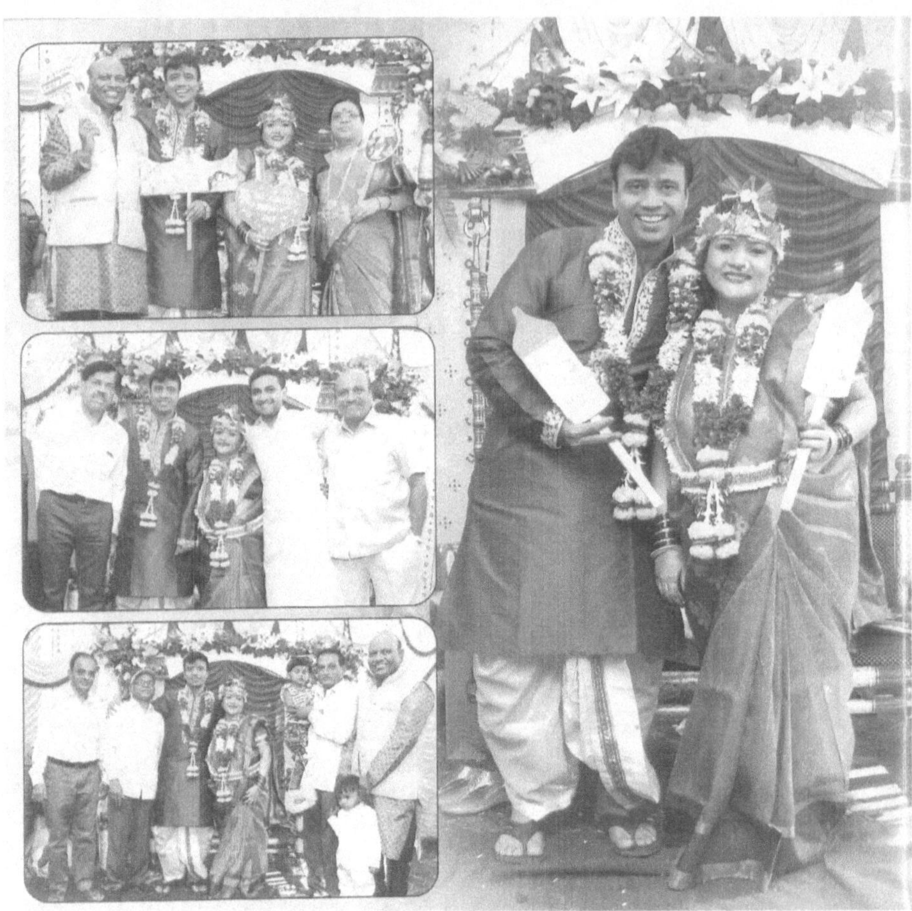

After a few days, we visited the doctor, and she informed us that we will have to operate and cannot wait for natural delivery considering that the baby was weighing on a higher side and I've had a miscarriage earlier.

We consulted the pandit and he gave us an auspicious day, 30th January for delivery. I was admitted on the 29th of January.

I couldn't sleep the whole night due to anxiety and worry. I harassed the nurse to keep checking my baby's heartbeat after every 2-3 hours. She understood my pain and worry so she religiously kept checking my baby's heartbeat.

I was assured that the baby was fine, and Naresh was with me the whole night. He didn't let me be alone even for a minute,.

The next morning arrived with a sense of urgency, as I was swiftly escorted to the operation theater. The clock seemed to taunt me with its relentless ticking, each passing second bringing me closer to a moment I could scarcely comprehend.

At 1 pm, on the 30th of January 2017, our baby girl, Yana, made her grand entrance into the world. As I held her fragile form in my arms, a flood of emotions overwhelmed me. Tears streamed down my cheeks, mingling with tears of joy and disbelief. At that moment, time stood still as I marveled at the miracle cradled in my arms.

It was a moment of sheer euphoria, a dream realized after enduring countless trials and tribulations. Despite the agony and anguish that had preceded this moment, there she was—our precious Yana—a symbol of hope and resilience in the face of adversity.

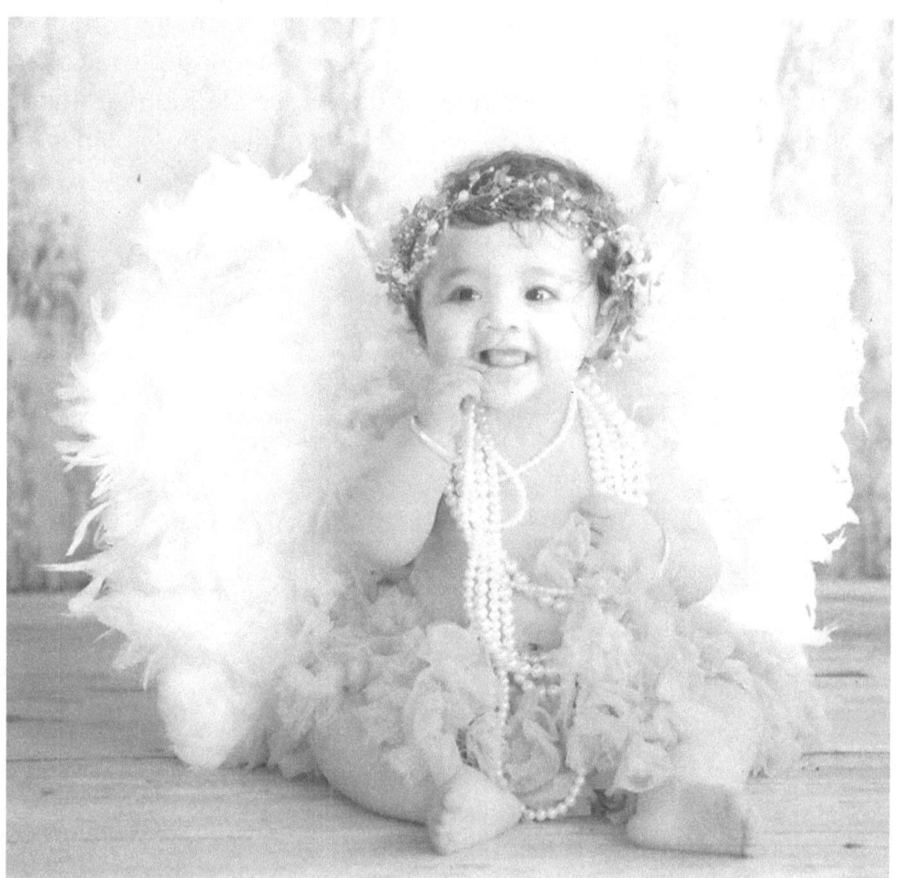

As I gazed into her innocent eyes, I knew that our journey had only just begun. But in that moment, as I held our daughter close, I felt an overwhelming sense of gratitude and triumph. Against all odds, against all the pain and uncertainty, we had emerged victorious. And in the warm glow of Yana's presence, I knew without doubt that we had won.

Upon returning home, my family orchestrated a grand welcome, a heartfelt celebration of love and anticipation for the newest member of our family, baby Yana. As I stepped through the threshold, the air was alive with excitement, and my heart swelled with joy at the sight before me.

Every corner of the room was adorned with vibrant flowers, their colors dancing in the soft glow of the evening light. The sweet fragrance of blooms filled the air, infusing the atmosphere with an aura of warmth and love.

As I took in the sight before me, my heart overflowed with gratitude for the love and support of my family. Their unwavering presence and boundless affection were a reminder of the incredible journey that lay ahead, filled with moments of joy, wonder, and endless possibilities.

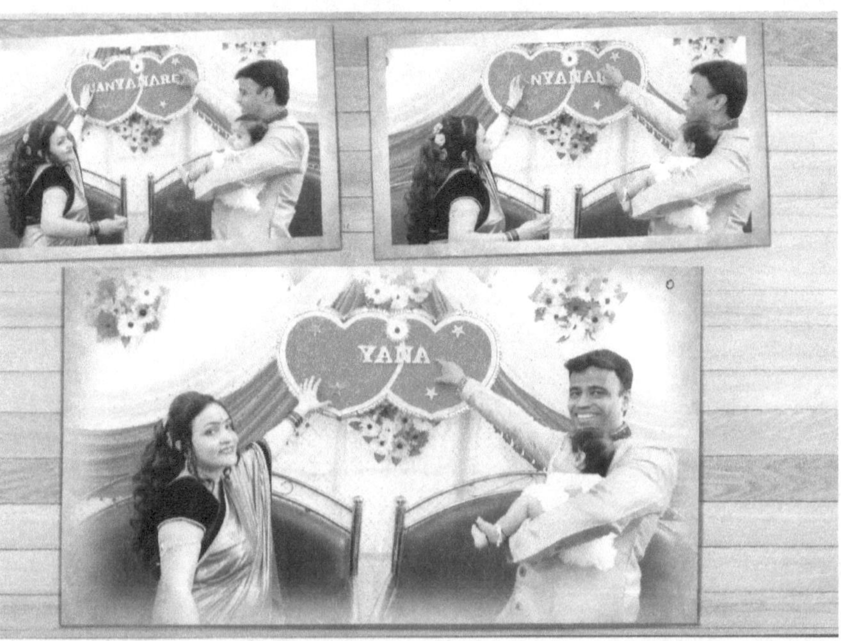

At that moment, surrounded by the beauty of love and anticipation, I knew that our family was ready to embark on this new chapter together. As I gazed upon the room, now transformed into a haven of love for our precious Yana, I felt a profound sense of peace and gratitude wash over me—a feeling that would stay with me for years to come.

Amidst the joy of Yana's arrival, life threw us another curveball. Just when everything seemed hale and hearty, we were struck by the devastating blow of losing my mother-in-law to cancer when Yana was just 9 months old. She was a pillar of strength, a beacon of hope, and her loss left a gaping hole in our hearts that no amount of time could ever fill.

Even in the face of her illness, my mother-in-law displayed remarkable courage, fighting with every ounce of strength she possessed until her last breath. I find solace in the fact that she had the opportunity to spend precious moments with Yana, her granddaughter. It was a bittersweet blessing, a fleeting ray of light in the darkness of our grief.

But with her passing, the weight of responsibility descended upon my shoulders like a crushing burden. Suddenly, the once-familiar rhythm of our lives was disrupted, replaced by the daunting task of managing the household single-handedly. In the absence of my mother-in-law, the void she left behind loomed large, a constant reminder of the irreplaceable loss we had endured.

Yet, amidst the chaos and upheaval, I found strength in the memory of her unwavering spirit. She had taught us the true meaning of resilience and perseverance, and I vowed to honor her legacy by carrying on in the face of adversity.

As I navigated the challenges of life without her guiding presence, I held onto the cherished memories we had shared, drawing comfort from the love that continued to surround us. Though the road ahead seemed daunting, I knew that her spirit would always be with us, guiding us through the darkest of days.

When Yana turned 11 months old, I joined the back office since business and work are my passion. My husband and father-in-law encouraged me to launch my own business in the field of corporate training, and I launched iFuture Technologies. I also joined the gym and started exercising regularly. Though I had delivered and achieved my goal, restarting the gym was high on my priority list because it was necessary for my overall health.

Despite the whirlwind of responsibilities that consumed my days—juggling work, managing the household, and caring for Yana—I couldn't shake the longing in my heart for another child. Deep down, I knew that the universe would grant my wish in due time.

My siblings and I share an unbreakable bond forged through years of shared laughter and tears. It was this bond, this sense of kinship and camaraderie, that fueled my desire for Yana to experience the joy of having a sibling of her own.

When Yana reached the tender age of two and a half, a whisper of intuition that had been building within me for some time, the signs were there—episodes of blackouts, a feeling of heaviness that hinted at the miracle unfolding within me.

After dropping Yana off at play group, with trembling hands, I purchased the pregnancy kit, my fingers fumbling as I tore open the packaging. And then, in a moment that felt suspended in time, I watched as two lines materialized before my eyes, confirming what my heart already knew.

Once again, I found myself overcome with that familiar rush of emotions. As I emerged from the confines of the washroom, clutching the pregnancy test in my hand, I couldn't contain the excitement bubbling within me.

With eager anticipation, I called my husband into the room, impatient to share the news that would undoubtedly change our lives once more. I extended the test towards him, and his eyes lit up with joy as he took in the sight before him.

Without a word, he kissed me gently on the forehead; his touch imbued with a warmth that filled me with reassurance and love. In that embrace, I found solace, knowing that no matter what lay ahead, we would face it together, hand in hand.

And then, with a smile that lit up his face, he pulled me close in a tight embrace, whispering those words that filled my heart with a sense of wonder and anticipation once more:

"Phir se baap banane wala hoon."

I shared the news with my siblings, and their excitement and support added to the overwhelming sense of joy that filled my heart. And then, with a heart full of anticipation, I called my mom to share the news, knowing that her love and wisdom would guide me through this new journey.

Everyone joined in the chorus of congratulations and well-wishes. In that moment, surrounded by love and support, I felt a sense of gratitude wash over me. Despite the challenges that lay ahead, I knew that I was not alone and that together, we would navigate this new chapter with joy and resilience.

Since my mother-in-law was not with me now. But my sisters and mother supported me unconditionally. This time fear didn't engulf me, I felt confident of delivering a healthy baby so, traveling to work, attending functions, and parties was pretty normal.

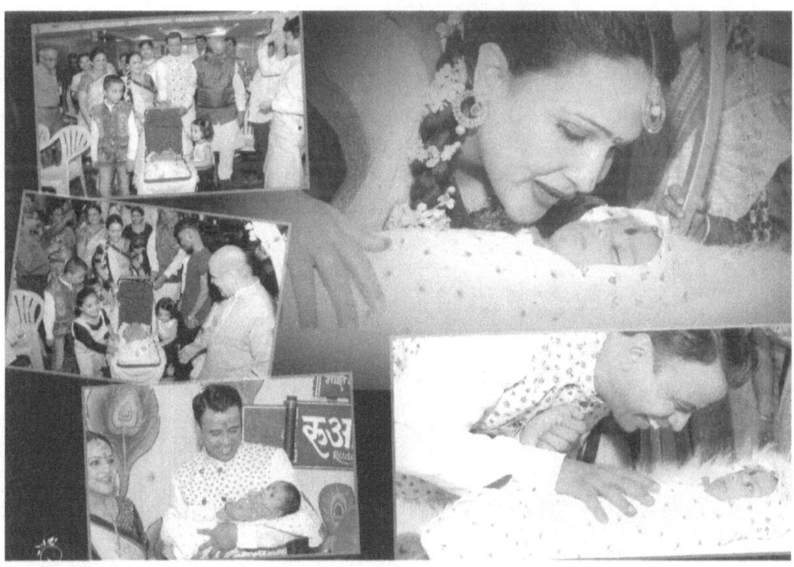

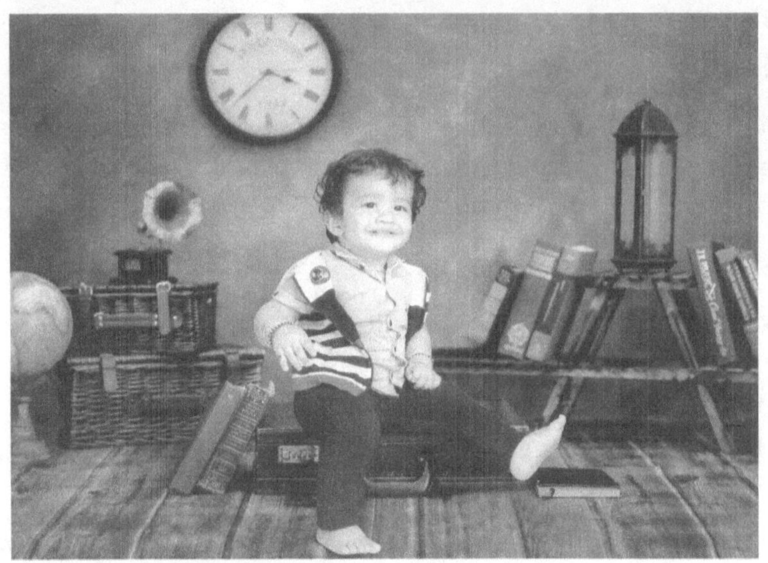

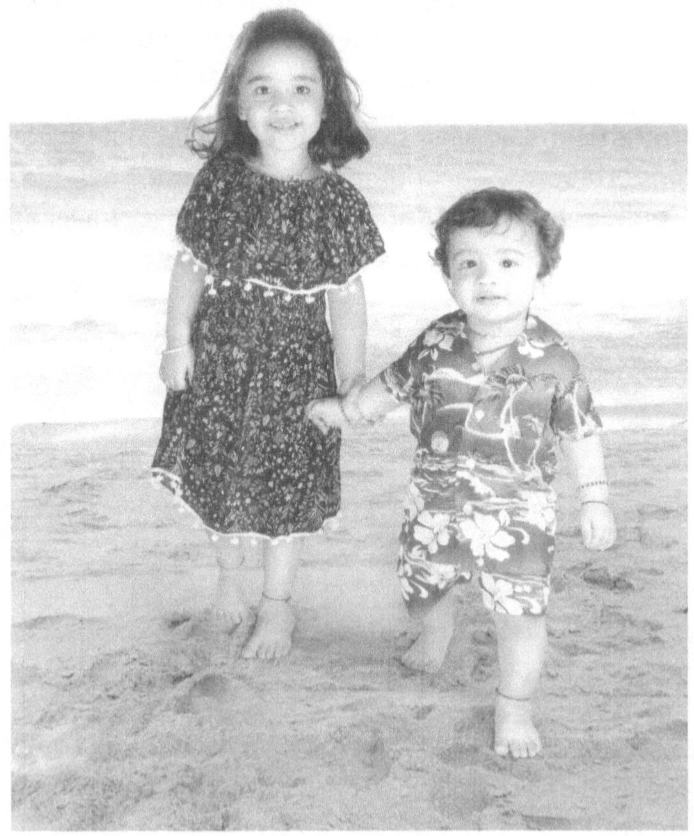

In March 2020, the world was hit by the COVID pandemic, disrupting lives and routines everywhere. However, despite the challenges posed by the pandemic, my commitment to my fitness journey remained steadfast. Determined to prioritize health and well-being, my husband and I decided to bring the gym to our home, investing in gym equipment and transforming our living space into a makeshift workout haven.

With resilience and determination, we embraced home workouts, delving into a variety of crossfit routines and cardio exercises to keep ourselves physically and mentally fit. Despite the uncertainties of the times, our dedication to maintaining a healthy lifestyle never wavered.

As the world gradually emerged from the grips of the pandemic, we made the decision to rejoin the gym, eager to resume our fitness journey in a familiar setting. The joy of returning to the gym, surrounded by like-minded individuals, reignited my passion for living a healthy life.

For me, prioritizing health is non-negotiable. Whether or not one chooses to have children is a deeply personal decision, but the importance of maintaining a healthy body, mind, and soul transcends individual choices. It is a commitment to oneself, a promise to nourish and care for the vessel that carries us through life's journey.

As I crossed the milestone of 40 years, my resolve to prioritize health only strengthened. Regular medical checkups have become a cornerstone of my wellness routine, ensuring that I remain proactive in safeguarding my health. Despite the sedentary nature of office life, I make a conscious effort to incorporate movement into my day, standing and conducting meetings to counteract the effects of prolonged sitting.

In essence, my journey towards living a healthy life is a testament to the resilience of the human spirit. It is a journey marked by determination, perseverance, and a deep-seated desire to give back to my body, mind, and soul the nourishment they deserve. And as I continue along this path, I am reminded that health is not just a destination, but a lifelong journey—one that I am committed to embracing wholeheartedly, every step of the way.

Minor lifestyle changes can indeed yield significant results. When aiming to lose weight or achieve any health goal, it's not necessary to adopt aggressive measures. Instead, consistency is key. Making small, sustainable changes and sticking to them diligently can make meaningful progress over time.

In my own journey, I experienced the power of gradual changes firsthand. After struggling with infertility and enduring a rollercoaster of emotions, I found solace in making lifestyle adjustments. Through regular exercise, mindful eating habits, and a holistic approach to wellness, I created an environment conducive to conception.

While assisted reproductive technologies like IVF are valuable options for many, they were not the right fit for me. Despite the disappointment of IVF not yielding the desired outcome, I remained steadfast in my belief that understanding and honoring my body's needs was paramount.

Ultimately, the key to a fulfilling life lies in self-awareness—knowing and respecting the intricate interplay of body, mind, and soul. By listening to our inner voice, nurturing our physical and emotional well-being, and embracing authenticity, we can embark on a journey of self-discovery and fulfillment.

In essence, "know thyself" serves as a guiding principle, reminding us to cultivate a deep understanding and appreciation for who we are. Through this journey of self-discovery, we unlock the potential to lead a life of purpose, balance, and harmony.

Despite the whirlwind of parenthood, my commitment to my fitness journey remains unwavering. I understand the importance of nurturing both body and mind, not just for myself but for the well-being of my loved ones.

With each passing day, I strive to lead by example, instilling in my children the value of a healthy lifestyle. Whether it's through daily exercise routines or mindful moments of reflection, I am dedicated to cultivating a nurturing environment where wellness is prioritized.

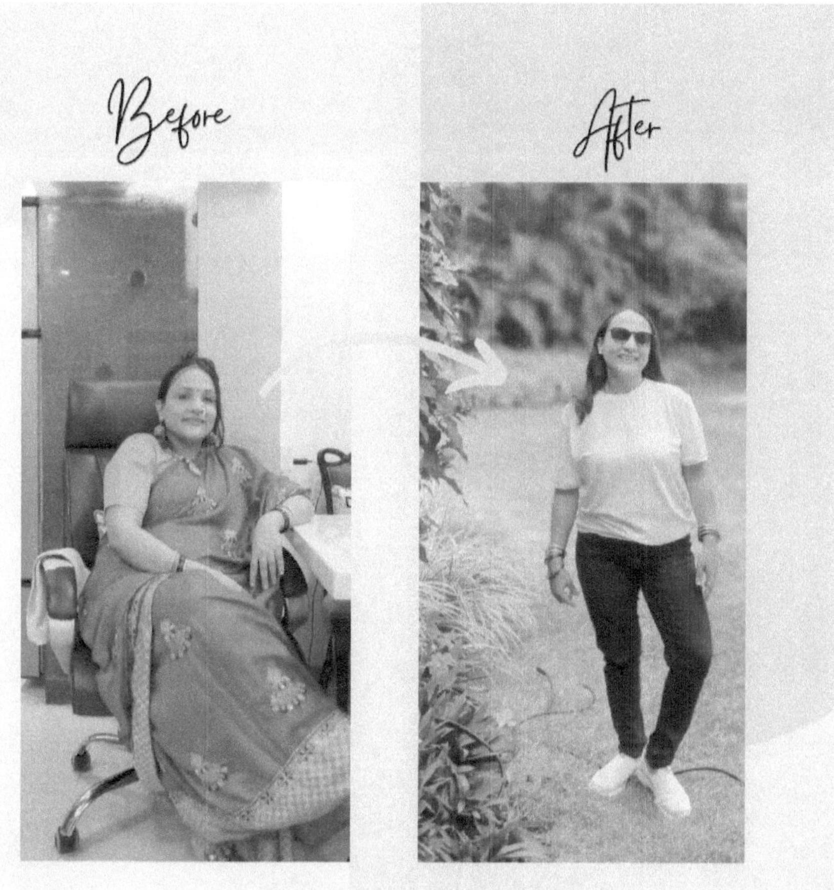

As I watch our children grow and thrive, I am reminded of the profound impact that a healthy body and mind can have on our lives. And so, my fitness journey continues, not just for myself, but for the ones I hold dear.

In the rhythm of our daily lives, amidst the laughter and chaos of parenthood, I find solace in knowing that we are building a foundation of health and happiness that will last a lifetime.